EAT TO SLEEP

1 3 5 7 9 10 8 6 4 2

Vermilion, an imprint of Ebury Publishing,
20 Vauxhall Bridge Road,
London SW1V 2SA

Vermilion is part of the Penguin Random House group of companies
whose addresses can be found at global.penguinrandomhouse.com

Penguin Random House UK

First published by Vermilion in 2018

www.penguin.co.uk

A CIP catalogue record for this book is available from the British Library

Design: Jim Smith
Project Editor: Victoria Marshallsay
Photography: Joff Lee
Food Styling: Mari Williams
Prop Styling: Joanna Harris

ISBN 9781785041839

Printed and bound in China by Toppan Leefung

EAT TO SLEEP

80 NOURISHING RECIPES TO HELP YOU SLEEP WELL EVERY NIGHT

HEATHER THOMAS
& ALINA TIERNEY, MSc

Vermilion

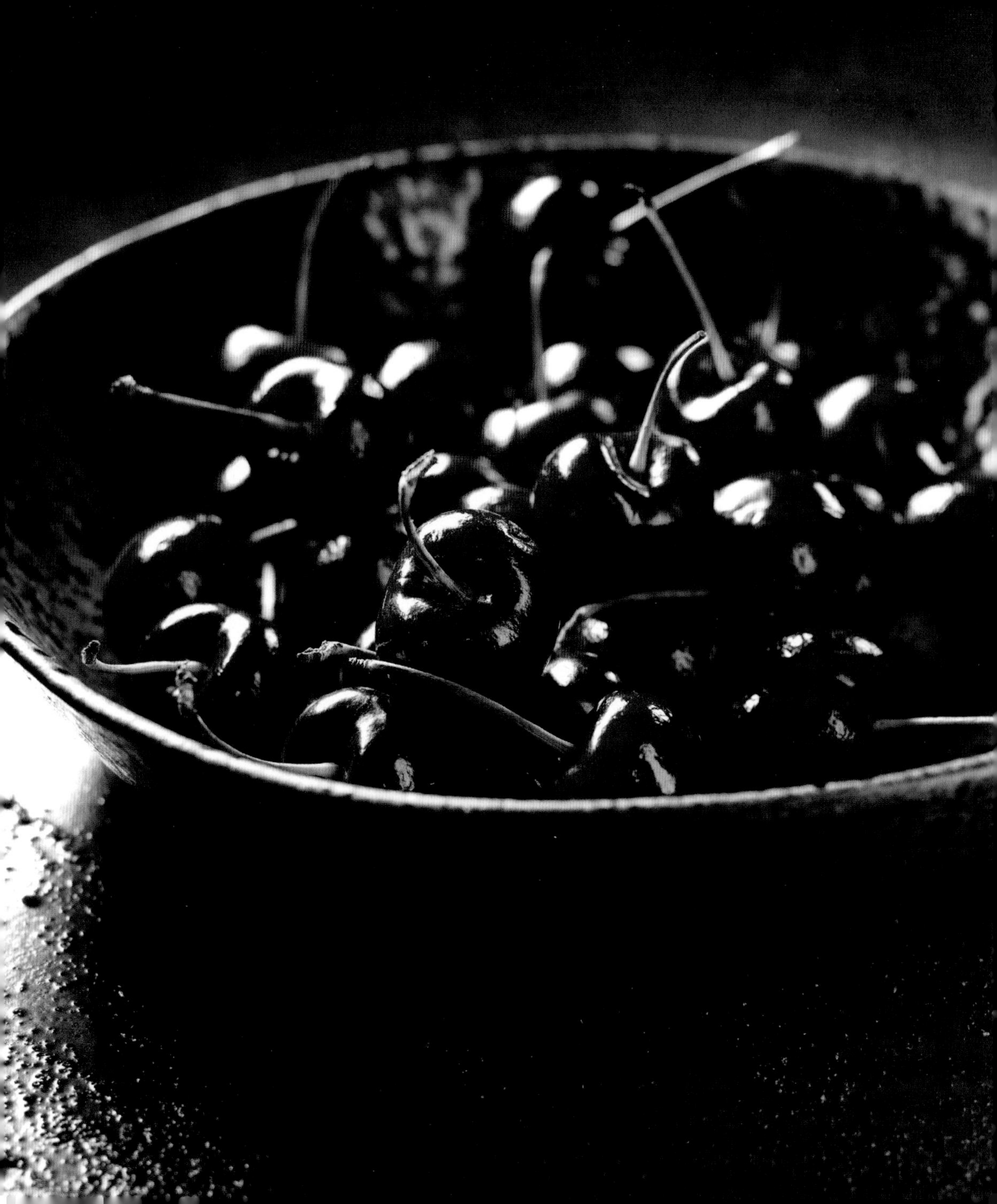

CONTENTS

Introduction

Sleep is just as important for our health as eating well and taking exercise; but the facts show that most of us are sleeping less, the quality of our sleep is deteriorating and insomnia is becoming increasingly common.

Growing awareness about the importance of sleep is starting to encourage us to understand how much sleep we get, how much we need, and how we can make positive and practical changes to sleep better. Many of us have sedentary jobs, don't exercise enough, have poor diets, and spend increasing time in front of computer, tablet and mobile phone screens – all of which are affecting the amount and quality of our sleep and, consequently, our health.

The good news is that it's possible to sleep longer and more soundly by making a few simple lifestyle changes, especially to our diets. If you struggle to get a good night's sleep, eating sleep-friendly foods and adjusting the timing of your meals could make a big difference. Sleep-friendly foods can calm your mind and boost the hormones that promote good sleep, helping to restore and repair your body while you rest.

This book features more than 80 delicious recipes to help you feel fitter, healthier and more energized, as well as sleep better so you are equipped to cope with the stresses of daily life.

How much sleep do you need?

To a great extent, the amount of sleep you need depends on your age: newborn babies need 14–17 hours, teenagers need 8–10 hours and, ideally, most adults should have eight hours a night.

However, everyone is different and the norm is in the region of seven to nine hours. One-third of us sleep only six hours or less and a poor night's sleep can be defined as less than five hours. As we get older, the length of time we sleep diminishes. Sleep can become disrupted by issues such as the increased need to urinate during the night or hot flushes during menopause.

The benefits of sleep

The health benefits of sleep are diverse and numerous. Sleep strengthens our immune system, helping to protect us from viruses and infections; lowers the risk of high blood pressure, heart disease, stroke and respiratory disorders; and reduces our risk of developing type 2 diabetes. Getting a good night's sleep on a regular basis is also important for enhancing and maintaining brain function, especially our memory, concentration, problem solving, performance and productivity.

The amount of sleep we get can also have an impact on inflammation in the body, especially in the gut and digestive system. There is some evidence that a correlation exists between sleep deprivation and inflammatory bowel diseases.

What makes us sleep?

Our circadian rhythm is the 24-hour internal clock that controls our sleep-wake cycle. It is aligned to the solar day and is affected by the hours of daylight and darkness. It is this system that regulates a number of neurotransmitters and hormones, such as serotonin and melatonin, that control when we sleep and when we are awake. Disruption of the sleep-wake cycle and deficiencies of these hormones are involved not only in sleep disorders but also in the pathology of mental health problems and depression. It is well known that a lack of serotonin is associated with depression and seasonal affective disorder (SAD).

The quality and physiology of our sleep is as important as the number of hours we average per night. If you are deprived of sleep and suffer from insomnia or periods of wakefulness, your sleep cycle will be interrupted, which can impact your health.

Sleep deprivation

Lack of sleep can lead to fatigue, loss of concentration and problems with memory and learning. Over the years there has been growing evidence to suggest that there is a link between little sleep and cardiovascular disease, type 2 diabetes, hypertension, respiratory disorders, obesity and other health conditions. Poor sleep patterns have also been linked to some mental health and emotional conditions, including difficulties with social interaction, anxiety, mood swings and depression.

How sleep affects weight

According to the US National Sleep Foundation, sleep deprivation can inhibit our ability to lose weight – even if we exercise regularly and eat healthily – increasing our risk of obesity, diabetes and cancer. This is because sleep deprivation affects the levels of the hormones (see pages 8–9) that regulate our appetites and consequently our food choices. Recent studies suggest that people who are sleep-deprived feel hungrier and crave food they don't need, especially refined carbohydrates and fats, making them more likely to gain weight. It is known that we consume fewer calories when we get good-quality sleep, helping us to maintain a healthy weight.

It's possible to sleep longer and more soundly by making a few simple lifestyle changes, especially to our diets.

Eating for sleep

The role of hormones

When it comes to getting a good night's sleep hormones play an important role. They help to maintain our sleep-wake cycle – making us feel sleepy in the evening and waking us up in the morning. By making a few small adjustments to your diet you can promote the hormones that have an impact on sleep.

Melatonin is a hormone that is essential for a healthy sleep cycle; it also controls the way we respond to stress. It's produced in the pineal gland in the brain when it becomes dark. When melatonin levels in the blood rise, sleep becomes inviting.

Bright and artificial light at night inhibits melatonin production, which is why it is advisable to avoid screens like TVs, laptops and phones just before bedtime. There are many other factors that can affect melatonin production, including smoking, stress, working night shifts, age and what you eat. If you are melatonin deficient, you may experience sleeplessness and insomnia.

Walnuts and cherries contain their own melatonin, so eating them may help you fall asleep more quickly. Oats, milk and bananas all boost our melatonin levels and can help to relieve insomnia – eating them regularly can help to stabilize your sleep cycle.

Serotonin is not found in food; it's a neurotransmitter derived from the amino acid tryptophan (see page 16). It plays an important role in regulating mood, appetite and sleeping as well as promoting feelings of calm and sleepiness; a deficiency of serotonin is linked to depression.

You can boost serotonin levels by eating tryptophan-rich foods (see page 16) with a side serving of complex carbs, such as oats or wholegrain bread. These carbs cause a slight spike in blood sugar and insulin levels, which helps the absorption of tryptophan into the brain, shortening the time it takes us to fall asleep. A glass of warm milk before going to bed can be a great idea – it contains small amounts of carbs (such as lactose) and also provides calcium and tryptophan that promote good levels of sleep-promoting serotonin and melatonin.

Key nutrients for sleep

The principal nutrients that help us nod off and experience quality sleep are:

- ★ Tryptophan
- ★ Vitamins B6 and D
- ★ Magnesium
- ★ Calcium
- ★ Potassium

In addition, there are many foods and herbs containing nutrients with sedative properties that can help to relax our nerves and muscles.

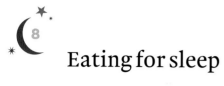

The following pages list the foods that will help you sleep more soundly. You can enjoy them in the 80 delicious recipes in this book.

How and when to eat

If you are experiencing problems with falling asleep, wakefulness and interrupted sleep, or waking up in the night with cramps, acid reflux or to go to the bathroom, it may be worth changing what you eat and the times at which you eat. This need not be a major dietary transformation – just tweaking what you eat for dinner and how you cook it, such as grilling, roasting and steaming which are kinder to your digestive system than frying. Also, aim not to eat too late – at least three hours before bed – to give yourself time to digest the food.

Sleep-friendly foods can calm the mind and boost the hormones that promote good sleep.

THE CYCLE OF POOR SLEEP

Cortisol influences a range of body systems and processes, including how we respond to stress, our immune response and metabolism. Levels of this hormone are usually high in the morning then decrease throughout the day, matching our activity and sleep patterns. If you lose a night's sleep, the following evening your cortisol levels will be elevated rather than lowered, making it more difficult for you to get to sleep, affecting the quality of your sleep and also increasing your appetite. If this occurs repeatedly, it can promote insulin resistance, increasing the risk of obesity.

High cortisol levels may also affect our food preferences, making us crave unhealthy foods that are higher in fat and/or sugar and making us more likely to snack. Research has shown that a high intake of caffeine (from coffee, tea, chocolate and soft drinks, including diet and energy drinks) raises cortisol levels, which can have an unhealthy effect on our ability to sleep and to manage stress, as well as causing headaches, rapid heart rate and irritability. Ideally, you should restrict your caffeine intake to a maximum of 400mg per day (the equivalent of four cups of brewed coffee) spread throughout the day or choose caffeine-free or decaf options if possible.

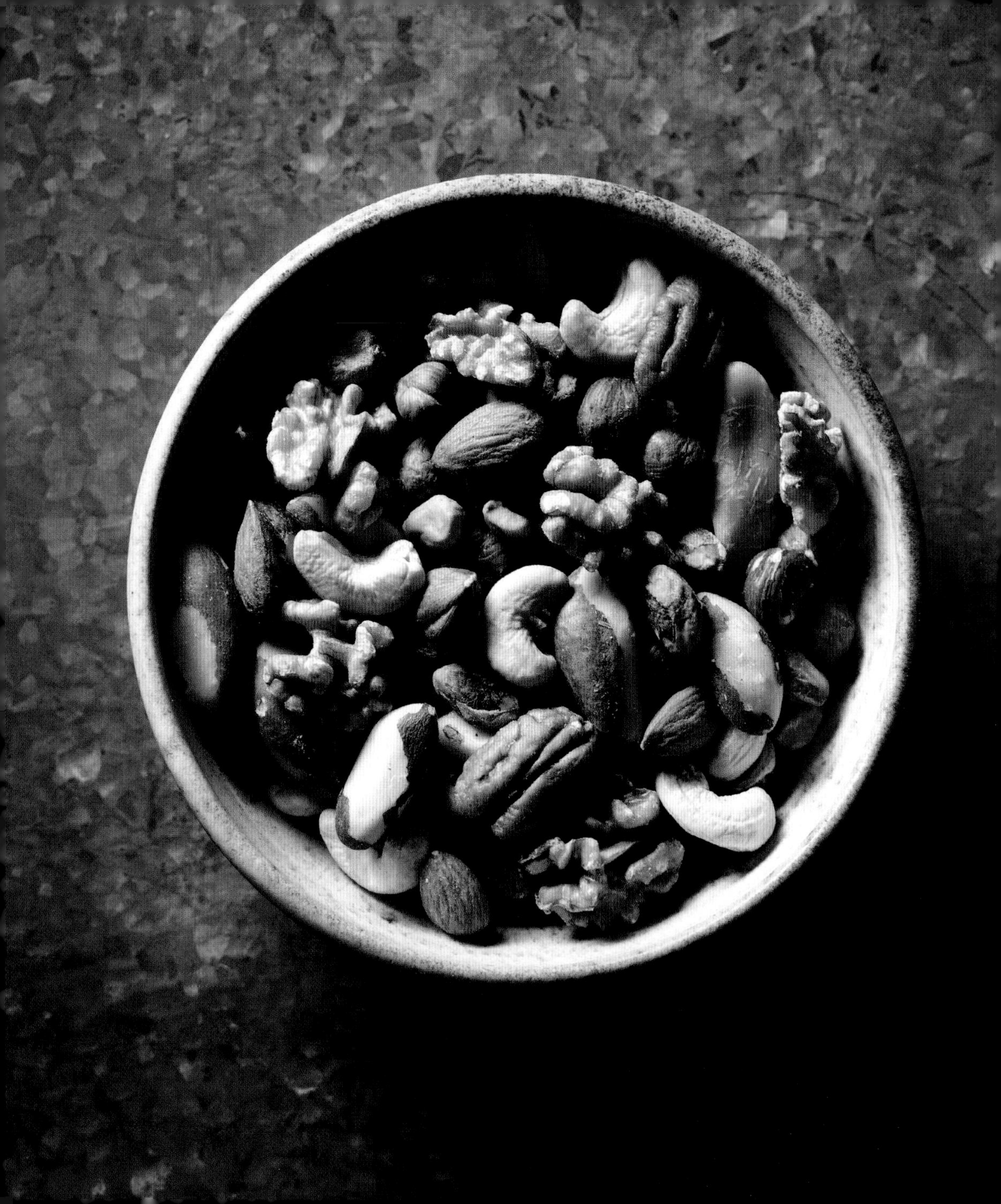

MAGNESIUM

This important mineral is needed for quality sleep and helps to activate the neurotransmitters that are responsible for calming your mind and body. It also helps muscles to relax, while steadying heart rhythm. Not having enough magnesium can cause sleep problems and even insomnia. Magnesium-rich foods include:

Nuts and seeds, especially almonds, Brazil nuts, cashews, pumpkin and sunflower seeds

Peanut butter

Bananas

Bulgur wheat

Barley

Brown rice

Oats and whole grains

Legumes and beans

Dark leafy green vegetables

Avocados

Yoghurt

Salmon

Mackerel

Dried fruit

Plain chocolate

CALCIUM

This helps the brain to use the amino acid tryptophan to make the sleep-inducing hormone melatonin and mood regulator serotonin. If you're calcium deficient, you might struggle to fall asleep. The benefits of a pre-bedtime mug of warm milk or some cheese and crackers are not old wives' tales – they really do work. Many foods are fortified with calcium, including soya milk, some breakfast cereals and bread. Calcium-rich foods include:

Nuts and seeds, especially almonds, hazelnuts, pistachios and sesame seeds

Cheese

Yoghurt

Milk

Sardines

Broccoli

Dark leafy green vegetables, especially kale and spinach

Figs

Seaweed

Beans, especially soya beans

Quinoa

VITAMIN B6

This vitamin plays an important role in the conversion of the sleep-enhancing amino acid tryptophan into serotonin – the neurotransmitter that stabilizes mood and aids healthy sleeping patterns. Foods containing vitamin B6 include:

Oily fish such as salmon and fresh tuna

Beef

Chicken

Offal

Wheat bran

Potatoes

Squash

Pistachios

Sunflower seeds

VITAMIN D

A deficiency in vitamin D may lead to sleep disruption in some people. Vitamin D is actually a hormone and not a vitamin and scientists think that it activates receptors in the brain that are associated with sleep. Getting plenty of fresh air is probably the best remedy of all, as sunlight promotes vitamin D synthesis in our skin. Foods containing vitamin D include:

Eggs

Oily fish such as sardines and salmon

Dairy products

Mushrooms

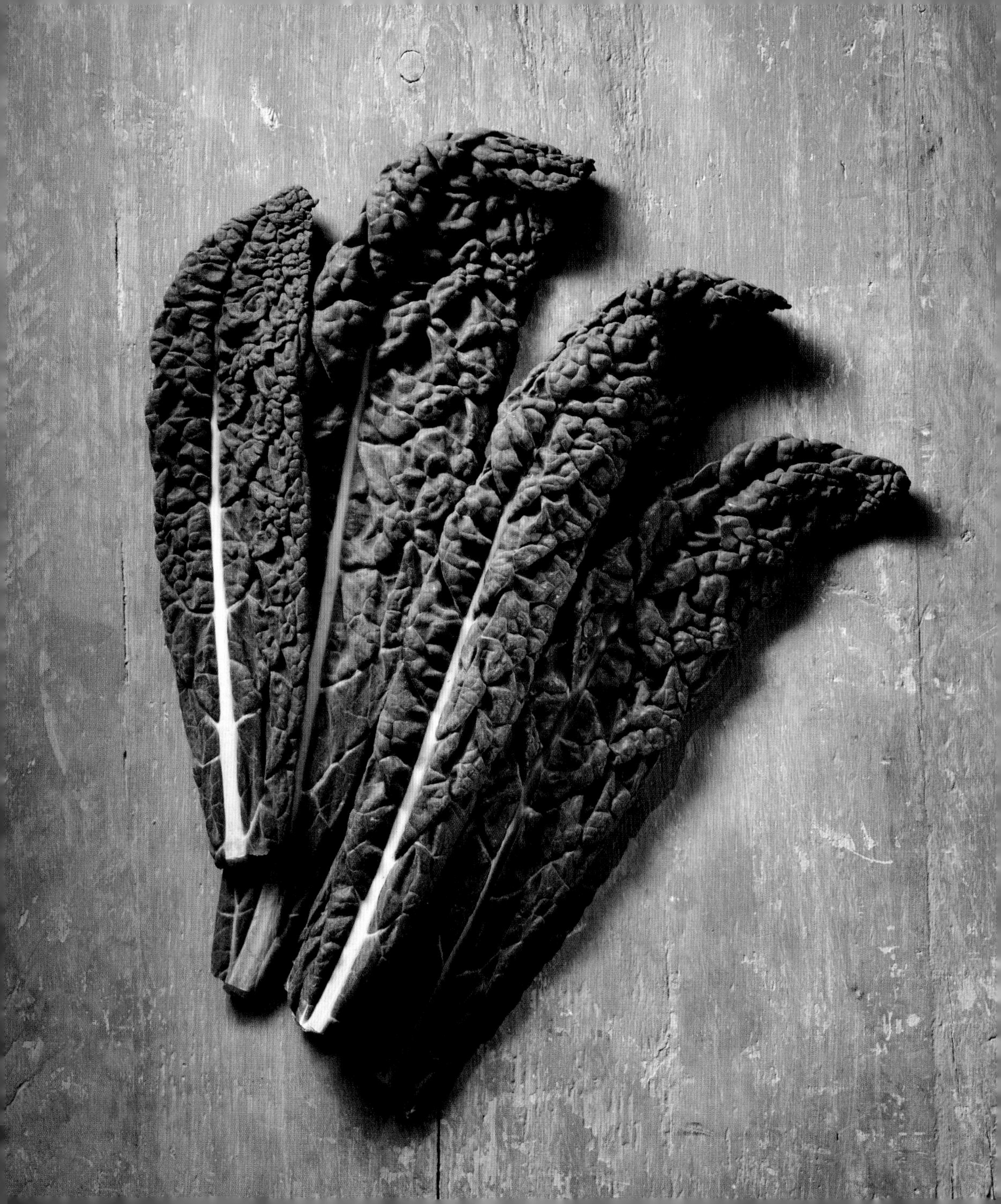

POTASSIUM

This is a muscle and nerve relaxant and aids good digestion. Too little potassium can lead to muscle spasms, which may disrupt your sleep. Potassium-rich foods include:

Sweet potatoes

Squash

Butterbeans

Edamame beans

Mushrooms

Dark leafy green vegetables

Potatoes

Watermelon

Beetroot

Papaya

Bananas

TRYPTOPHAN

This regulates our moods, calms us, fights anxiety, and has a natural sedative effect. It's an essential amino acid (a building block of protein), which means that our bodies can't make it and we have to obtain it from food. Its main function is to serve as a precursor to serotonin, melatonin and niacin (vitamin B3). Lean proteins are high in tryptophan and easy to digest. Tryptophan-rich foods are:

Fish

Chicken

Turkey

Nuts and seeds, especially almonds and walnuts

Cheese

Milk

Yoghurt

Soy products

Whole grains

Oats

Quinoa

Brown rice

Beans

Lentils

Bananas

Potatoes

GLYCINE

This is a mild sedative and nerve and muscle relaxant that can help to induce sleepiness and promote restful sleep. Like tryptophan, glycine is an amino acid, but unlike tryptophan, it is non essential (that means the body can produce it itself). Consuming glycine before bedtime significantly improves sleep quality for those with insomniac tendencies. Glycine-rich foods include:

Chamomile

Passionflower

Lemon balm tea and tisanes

Home-made beef and chicken broth

Dairy products

Fish

Meat

Dark leafy green vegetables

Sleep-inhibiting foods

If you want a good night's sleep, try to avoid consuming the foods listed below late in the day. They are more likely to stimulate you and keep you wide awake than send you to sleep.

Artificial sweeteners might be sugar free and lower in calories, but there is evidence to suggest that they may adversely affect sleep. If you need to sweeten drinks and desserts, use raw honey (honey is soothing and can be conducive to sleep as it enables tryptophan to enter the brain).

Simple carbohydrates are quickly broken down into sugar molecules and can have a major effect on blood glucose levels. Try to avoid over-refined simple carbs and sugary foods such as white bread, pasta, pastry, cookies, cakes and sweets before going to bed, as these can lead to significant spikes in blood glucose levels. High blood sugar levels during the night may increase your need to go to the toilet and make you feel too warm or unsettled. Check the sugar content on the labels of sauces, ready meals and snacks. Look out for 'hidden' sugars too, including corn syrup, fructose, sucrose, dextrose, maltose, glucose, rice syrup, caramel and sorbitol.

Monosodium glutamate (MSG) is a commonly used food additive found in many refined foods and Chinese dishes. It is a brain stimulant and has been linked to night-time wakefulness. Check the labels when buying soy sauce and packaged foods. MSG is also used as a flavour enhancer by many fast food outlets, so check with the staff.

Alcohol is both a stimulant and a depressant; it can cause you to sleep fitfully, feel dehydrated, experience a headache and feel tired. If you drink regularly most evenings, you are more likely to be affected by insomnia.

Coffee, tea and caffeinated soft drinks stimulate your nervous system and keep you awake by blocking the effects of adenosine, a neuro-transmitter that signals to the brain that it is time to rest. The stimulatory effect of caffeine lasts for at least 8–12 hours after consumption, so it's sensible to avoid it from early afternoon onward. In addition, caffeine is a natural diuretic, so it stimulates the need to get up and urinate during the night.

Chocolate, especially milk chocolate, contains sugar and fat as well as caffeine from the cocoa beans. It also contains other stimulants, including theobromine, which raises the heart rate and causes insomnia. If you really can't do without chocolate in the evening, stick to the bitter plain sort (at least 70% cocoa solids), which contains magnesium but very little sugar, and eat it only in moderation and not too late. White chocolate, which is theobromine free, is lower in caffeine and more likely to be tolerated in small quantities, but watch out for the sugar content which can be almost 50%.

Spicy foods can worsen acid reflux and cause gastrointestinal discomfort in some people. It may be sensible to limit the amount of spicy food you eat before going to bed and to opt for blander, more soothing alternatives.

Tomatoes eaten in large amounts at dinner time may cause heartburn and indigestion in some people due to their high acid content.

Processed meats, including bacon, ham and pepperoni, contain high levels of sodium and can disrupt sleep by raising your blood pressure, so they are best avoided in the evening.

Fatty and fried foods are best avoided in the evening. They can cause indigestion, which can lead to wakefulness in the night.

The stimulatory effect of caffeine lasts for at least 8–12 hours after consumption, so it's sensible to avoid it from early afternoon onwards.

GUIDELINES TO HELP YOU SLEEP

- ★ **Don't** eat a big meal close to bedtime, especially if you tend to get indigestion. Eat early, preferably three hours or more before going to bed and don't over-indulge. Over-eating will make it more difficult for your body to digest the food.
- ★ **Don't** drink caffeinated drinks late in the day. As caffeine is a stimulant, it will make it harder for you to get to sleep and may cause night wakefulness. It is also a diuretic, stimulating urination and reducing hydration.
- ★ **Don't** eat food stimulants such as chillies, spicy dishes and processed meats.
- ★ **Don't** drink too much alcohol, especially in the evening. It may be relaxing, but its effects soon wear off and lead to wakefulness in the small hours.
- ★ **Don't** consume too many fluids before going to bed. Although you need to be well hydrated, you don't want to be waking up regularly to visit the bathroom and then experience problems going back to sleep.
- ★ **Do** eat foods that will help induce sleep.
- ★ **Do** eat enough calories during the day so that you don't feel hungry in the night.
- ★ **Do** have a soothing hot milky drink or herbal tisane at bedtime.

1

LIGHT SUPPERS

Crunchy prawn and rice noodle salad

SERVES 4
PREP: 15 minutes
COOK: 2 minutes

225 g/8 oz thin rice noodles (dry weight)
250 g/9 oz mangetout, trimmed
1 red pepper, deseeded and thinly sliced
1 yellow pepper, deseeded and thinly sliced
2 carrots, cut into thin matchsticks
85 g/3 oz bean sprouts
1 bunch spring onions, sliced
450 g/1 lb peeled cooked large prawns
1 ripe avocado, stoned, peeled and cubed
1 small bunch fresh coriander, chopped
60 g/2 oz crushed salted peanuts

FOR THE DRESSING:
2 tbsp Thai fish sauce
1 tbsp light soy sauce
juice of 2 limes
1 tbsp light brown sugar
1 tbsp sweet chilli sauce
1 garlic clove, crushed

This delicious crunchy salad is so quick and easy to prepare. Prawns contain tryptophan which is calming and sedating, and rice noodles are easier to digest than wheat or egg ones that contain gluten.

Put the noodles in a heatproof shallow bowl and pour boiling water over them. Cover with cling film and set aside for about 5 minutes until they are just tender but not too soft. Drain, leave to cool and then pat dry with kitchen paper.

Meanwhile, add the mangetout to a pan of boiling water and cook for about 2 minutes until just tender. Drain and refresh immediately in a bowl of iced water. Drain and pat dry with kitchen paper, then cut each one diagonally into 2–3 pieces.

Mix the mangetout with the peppers, carrots, bean sprouts, spring onions, prawns, avocado, coriander and drained noodles.

Put all the ingredients for the dressing in a bowl and stir well until combined. Alternatively, shake in a screw-top jar.

Toss the noodles and vegetables in the dressing and divide between four serving plates. Scatter the peanuts over the top and serve.

Or you can try this ...

★ Use sugar snap peas instead of mangetout.
★ Add some rocket, watercress or steamed pak choi.
★ Use shredded cooked chicken or rare roast beef instead of prawns.

Warm salmon and quinoa salad

Quinoa is a great source of vegetable protein and dietary fibre and is gluten-free. It also contains calcium, which helps your brain use tryptophan to make melatonin.

SERVES 4
PREP: 15 minutes
COOK: 15 minutes

- 4 x 150 g/5 oz skinned salmon fillets
- 250 g/9 oz quinoa (dry weight)
- 2 tbsp olive oil, plus extra for brushing
- 2 courgettes, thinly sliced lengthwise
- grated zest and juice of 1 lemon
- 120 g/4 oz frozen soya beans, defrosted
- 1 small bunch spring onions, thinly sliced
- 1 tbsp chia seeds
- 1 tbsp sesame seeds
- a handful of dill, chopped
- salt and freshly ground black pepper
- 225 g/8 oz tzatziki to serve

Preheat the oven to 180°C/350°F/gas 4.

Place the salmon fillets on a large piece of kitchen foil and fold it over loosely to make a parcel, sealing the edges. Place on a baking sheet and cook in the preheated oven for about 15 minutes until the salmon is cooked through. Remove from the foil and cut into large flakes.

Meanwhile, cook the quinoa according to the instructions on the packet.

Lightly brush a ridged griddle pan with oil and set over a medium heat. Add the courgette slices to the hot pan, a few at a time, and cook for about 2 minutes each side until just tender and attractively striped.

Stir the olive oil, lemon zest and juice into the quinoa. Mix in the soya beans, spring onions, seeds and most of the dill. Season to taste and divide between four serving plates.

Top with the salmon and griddled courgette strips, then sprinkle with the remaining dill. Serve immediately with the tzatziki.

Or you can try this…

★ Instead of soya beans, use canned flageolets or kidney beans.
★ Add some griddled fennel bulb, aubergine or sweet peppers.
★ Instead of the tzatziki, serve with some sliced avocado or a drizzle of pesto.

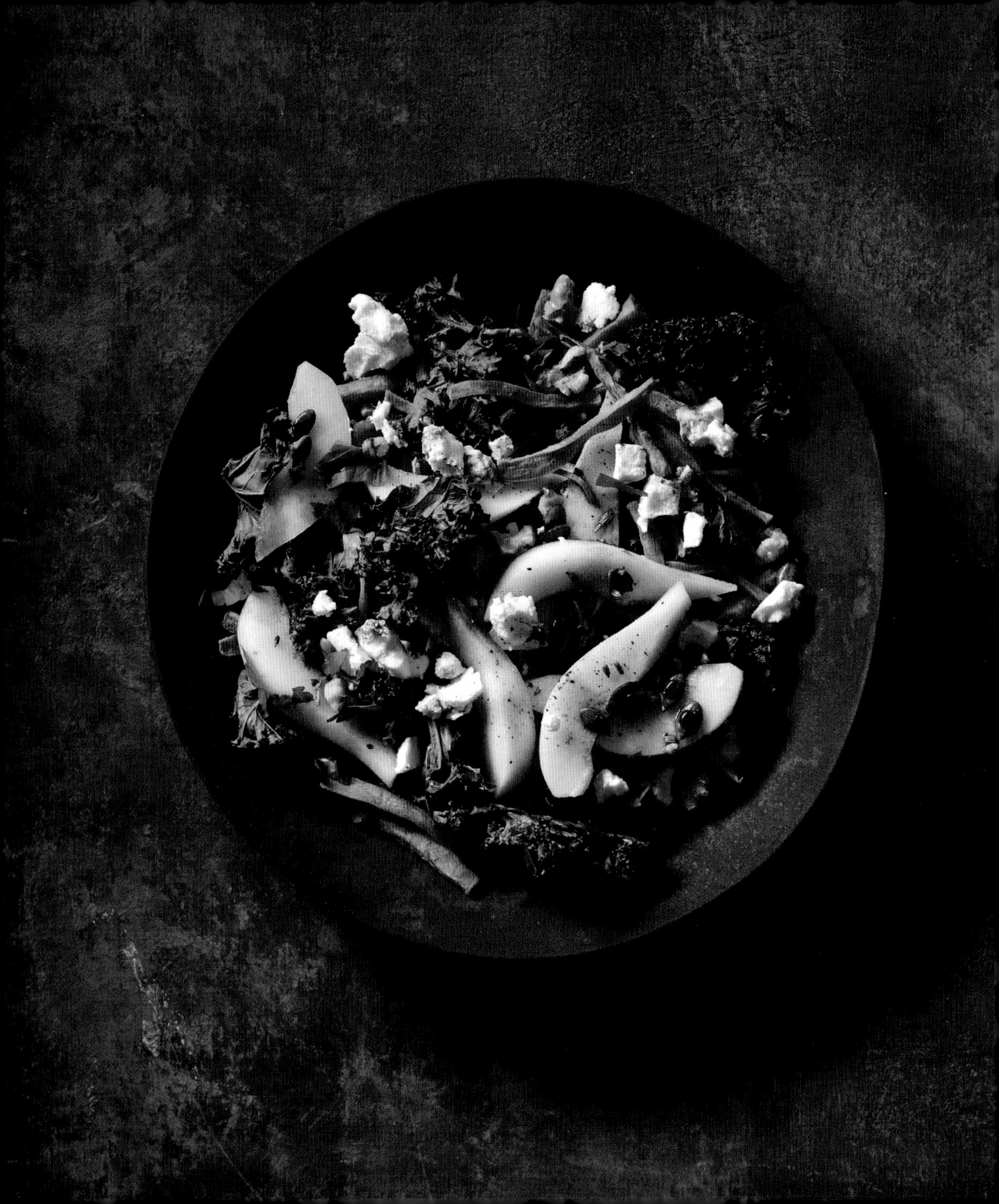

Warm roasted kale, pear and sweet potato salad

This warm salad is a jackpot of sleep-friendly nutrients. The kale and seeds provide calcium and magnesium; the sweet potatoes are a good source of potassium and vitamin B6 and the goats' cheese has vitamin D.

SERVES 4
PREP: 15 minutes
COOK: 25 minutes

2 large sweet potatoes, peeled and cut into thick matchsticks
4 tbsp olive oil
60 g/2 oz mixed seeds, e.g. cumin, fennel and pumpkin seeds
300 g/10 oz kale, ribs and stalks removed, leaves coarsely shredded
60 g/2 oz chopped walnuts
175 g/6 oz creamy goats' cheese, crumbled
2 ripe pears, peeled, cored and sliced
4 tsp balsamic vinegar
a handful of fresh flat-leaf parsley, finely chopped
salt and freshly ground black pepper

Preheat the oven to 190°C/375°F/gas mark 5.

Put the sweet potato in a large roasting pan and sprinkle with the oil. Season lightly with salt and pepper. Bake in the preheated oven for about 8 minutes, then sprinkle the seeds over the top and return to the oven for 5 minutes.

Add the kale and stir it gently into the seedy oil. Roast for 8–10 minutes until the sweet potato is tender and the kale is crisp but not browned. Remove from the oven and stir in the walnuts.

Divide the roasted vegetable mixture between four serving plates. Crumble the goats' cheese over the top and add the pears. Drizzle with balsamic vinegar, sprinkle with parsley and serve warm.

Or you can try this …

★ Use feta or Gorgonzola instead of goats' cheese.
★ Use butternut squash instead of sweet potatoes.
★ Stir some lentils into the salad to make it more substantial.

Fruity coleslaw in seedy yoghurt dressing

SERVES 4–6
PREP: 20 minutes
COOK: 5 minutes

60 g/2 oz shelled pistachios
2 tbsp pine nuts
1 small red cabbage, cored and finely shredded
200 g/7 oz kale, ribs and stalks removed, leaves shredded
1 red onion, coarsely grated
2 carrots, coarsely grated
6 medjool dates, chopped
2 ruby red grapefruit, cut into segments
a handful of fresh flat-leaf parsley, chopped
a handful of fresh coriander, chopped
juice of 1 orange
a large pinch of ground cinnamon

FOR THE DRESSING:
2 tbsp olive oil
2.5 cm/1 in piece fresh root ginger, peeled and diced
1 tbsp black mustard seeds
1 tbsp nigella seeds
1 tsp cumin seeds
150 g/5 oz 0% fat Greek yoghurt
salt and freshly ground black pepper

This coleslaw almost makes a meal in itself and contains a wealth of nutrients to help you sleep. Serve it with griddled chicken or as a great topping for baked jacket potatoes or sweet potatoes.

Place a small frying pan over a medium heat and toast the pistachios and pine nuts for 1–2 minutes, tossing gently, until golden brown. Remove from the pan and cool.

Put the red cabbage, kale, onion, carrots, dates, grapefruit segments and herbs in a large serving bowl. Sprinkle with the orange juice and cinnamon.

Make the dressing: heat the oil in a pan set over a low heat. Add the ginger and seeds and cook for 1–2 minutes until they release their aroma. Remove from the heat and stir in the yoghurt. Season to taste with salt and pepper.

Pour the dressing over the salad and toss gently until everything is lightly coated. Sprinkle with the toasted pistachios and pine nuts and serve.

Or you can try this …

★ Use a white cabbage and some finely chopped spring onions instead of the red cabbage and kale.
★ Use lemon instead of orange juice.
★ Mix 1–2 tablespoons of light mayonnaise into the yoghurt dressing.
★ Sprinkle the coleslaw with ruby red pomegranate seeds.

Chicken, bulgur wheat and broccoli salad

Low magnesium levels can impair the quality of your sleep and bulgur wheat is a good source of this vital mineral.

SERVES 4
PREP: 15 minutes
COOK: 20 minutes

- oil for brushing
- 3 boned chicken breasts
- 200 g/7 oz bulgur wheat (dry weight)
- 240 ml/8 fl oz vegetable stock
- 400 g/14 oz tenderstem broccoli, trimmed and each stalk cut in half
- 120 g/4 oz mixed sprouted seeds, e.g. alfalfa, broccoli or radish
- 1 avocado, stoned, peeled and thinly sliced
- 150 g/5 oz soft creamy goats' cheese, cut into pieces
- 1 small bunch fresh chives, snipped
- salt and freshly ground black pepper

FOR THE VINAIGRETTE:

- 2 tbsp black and/or white sesame seeds
- 3 tbsp sunflower oil
- 1 tbsp toasted sesame oil
- 2 tbsp rice vinegar
- 2 tbsp light soy sauce
- juice of 1 lime
- 1 garlic clove, finely chopped
- 1 tsp grated fresh root ginger
- 1 tbsp clear honey

Make the sesame honey vinaigrette: toast the sesame seeds in a dry frying pan set over a medium heat for 2–3 minutes, shaking gently, until golden brown. Remove immediately and when cool place with the remaining dressing ingredients in a screw-top jar. Shake until well combined.

Lightly oil a griddle pan and set over a medium to high heat. Add the chicken breasts to the hot pan and cook for about 15 minutes, turning halfway through, until golden brown and thoroughly cooked. Cut into thin slices.

Meanwhile, put the bulgur wheat and stock in a saucepan and bring to the boil. Reduce the heat, cover the pan and simmer for 5 minutes. Remove from the heat and leave, covered, for at least another 5 minutes or until the grains are tender and have absorbed most or all of the stock.

Steam the broccoli in a steamer or a colander placed over a saucepan of simmering water for about 5 minutes until it's just tender but still retains a little 'bite'.

Mix the bulgur wheat with the sprouted seeds, avocado and warm broccoli in a large bowl. Add the dressing and toss gently, seasoning to taste with salt and pepper.

Divide the salad between four serving plates and dot with the goats' cheese. Top with the sliced chicken and sprinkle with chives.

Superfood salad

SERVES 4
PREP: 15 minutes
COOK: 2 minutes

225 g/8 oz kale, ribs and stalks removed, leaves shredded
2 tbsp pumpkin seeds
85 g/3 oz cashews
1 large courgette, cut into matchsticks
2 carrots, coarsely grated or cut into thin strips with a potato peeler
4 spring onions, sliced
225 g/8 oz edamame beans, cooked or frozen and defrosted
150 g/5 oz mixed sprouted seeds, e.g. amaranth, alfalfa, broccoli, radish, pea or bean sprouts
1 ripe avocado, stoned, peeled and cubed
1 small bunch fresh flat-leaf parsley, chopped
120 g/4 oz feta cheese

FOR THE DRESSING:
4 tbsp olive oil
2 tbsp cider vinegar
1 tbsp grated fresh root ginger
1 garlic clove, crushed
grated zest and juice of 1 orange
1 tsp clear honey
2 tbsp sesame seeds
salt and freshly ground black pepper

Salads don't get much more nutritious than this one. Dark green leafy vegetables, such as kale, are great to eat in the evening because they contain glycine, a mild sedative and nerve and muscle relaxant.

Blanch the kale by adding it to a saucepan of boiling salted water. Cook for 30 seconds and then drain well in a colander.

Toast the pumpkin seeds and cashews in a dry frying pan set over a medium heat for 1–2 minutes, tossing gently, until golden brown. Remove immediately and set aside to cool.

Put the warm kale in a bowl with the courgette, carrots, spring onions, edamame beans, sprouts and avocado. Stir in the parsley and toasted seeds and cashews.

Make the dressing: mix all the ingredients together until thoroughly combined.

Pour the dressing over the salad and toss gently. Crumble the cheese over the top and serve immediately.

Or you can try this...

★ Add some sliced fennel bulb or red or yellow peppers.
★ Walnuts, pecans, hazelnuts, pistachios or almonds can be substituted for the cashews.
★ Make the salad sweet by adding diced apple, pear, mango or pomegranate seeds.
★ Vary the beans: try chickpeas or butterbeans.

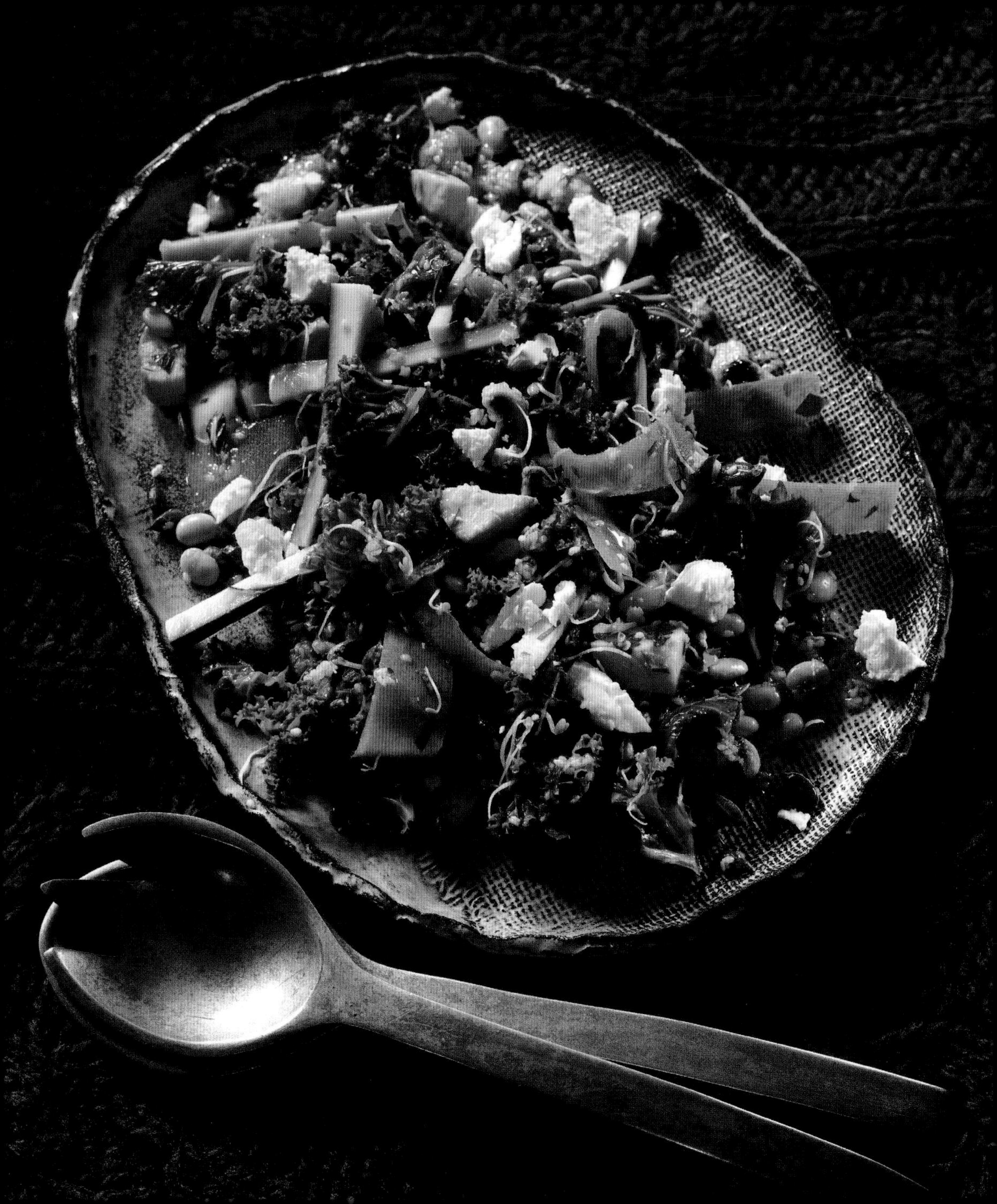

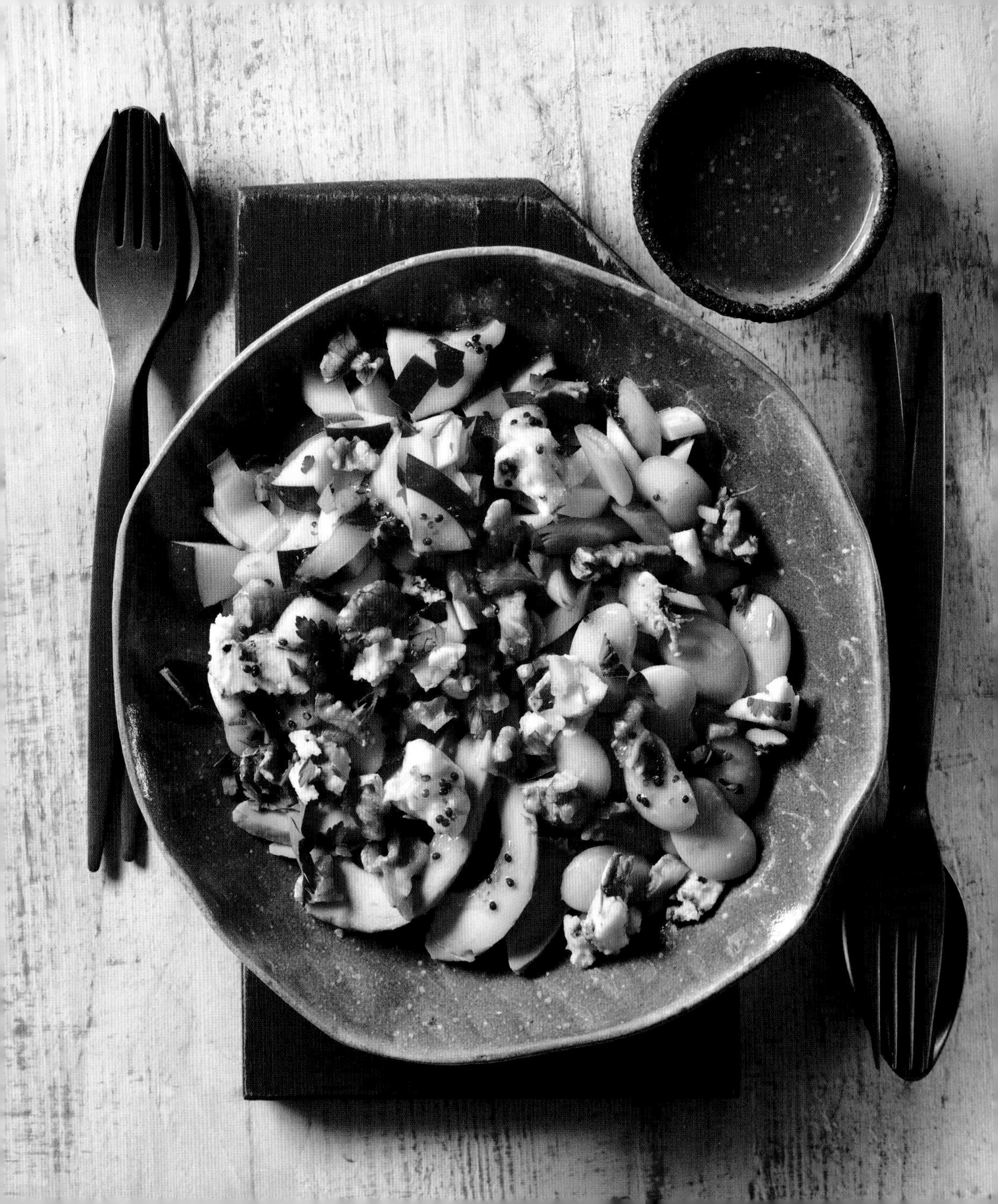

Butterbean, chicory and avocado salad

Combining sweet and savoury tastes is always a winner, especially as an accompaniment for cold meat, poultry and game. Avocados contain magnesium, potassium and vitamin B6, which all help to induce sleep.

SERVES 4
PREP: 15 minutes

3 heads white or red chicory
2 red apples
1 bunch spring onions, finely chopped
1 ripe avocado, stoned, peeled and sliced
1 x 400 g/14 oz can butterbeans, rinsed and drained
120 g/4 oz Roquefort cheese, diced or crumbled
60 g/2 oz chopped walnuts
1 small bunch fresh flat-leaf parsley, finely chopped

FOR THE HONEY MUSTARD VINAIGRETTE:
4 tbsp olive oil
1 tbsp cider vinegar
2 tsp honey mustard
juice of 1 lemon
salt and freshly ground black pepper

Trim the fat bases off the chicory and thinly slice the heads into rounds. Core the apples and cut them into small cubes.

Mix the chicory, apples, spring onions, avocado, butterbeans, Roquefort, walnuts and parsley in a bowl.

Make the honey mustard vinaigrette: blend the oil and vinegar with the honey mustard and lemon juice and season to taste with salt and pepper.

Pour the dressing over the chicory salad and toss gently together. Serve immediately.

Or you can try this …

- ★ Use diced or sliced pears instead of apples, or even stoned lychees.
- ★ Vary the beans: try kidney beans, flageolets or even some blanched crunchy fine green beans.
- ★ Make this salad more substantial by serving it with chicken.

Chicken and chickpea wraps

SERVES 4
PREP: 20 minutes
COOK: 10–12 minutes

675 g / 1½ lb boneless skinned chicken breast fillets
1 x 400 g / 14 oz can chickpeas, drained and rinsed
2 garlic cloves, crushed
3 tbsp olive oil
a squeeze of lemon juice
1 tbsp cumin seeds, crushed
4 large seedy wholemeal wraps
Greek yoghurt or labneh to serve

FOR THE MARINADE:
1 tsp sumac
½ tsp ground cumin
½ tsp ras el hanout
½ tsp ground turmeric
a pinch each of ground cinnamon and cardamom
grated zest and juice of ½ lemon
3 tbsp olive oil
2 garlic cloves, crushed
a handful of fresh coriander, chopped

FOR THE AVOCADO SALAD:
1 medium avocado, stoned, peeled and diced
½ red onion, diced
1 large bunch fresh coriander, finely chopped
juice of ½ lemon
salt and freshly ground black pepper

Chicken and chickpeas are a great combination – they both contain vitamin B6 and tryptophan, while avocado is a good source of magnesium and potassium, which relax your muscles and aid quality sleep.

Make the marinade: dry-fry all the spices in a small frying pan for 1–2 minutes until they release their aroma. Tip them into a large bowl and stir in the remaining ingredients. Add the chicken and marinate for at least 30 minutes (overnight in the fridge if you like).

Meanwhile, coarsely mash the chickpeas with the garlic, olive oil, lemon juice and cumin seeds. Season lightly with salt and pepper.

Mix all the ingredients for the avocado salad in a bowl and set aside.

When you're ready to cook the chicken, heat a large heavy-based frying pan or ridged griddle pan over a medium to high heat. When it's hot, add the chicken and cook for about 10 minutes, turning occasionally, until golden brown on the outside and cooked right through inside. Remove from the pan and allow it to rest for a few minutes before slicing thinly.

Heat the wraps in a large frying pan set over a low heat or in a low oven. Spread with the mashed chickpeas and top with the avocado salad and the chicken. Roll up or fold over and eat warm with some yoghurt or labneh.

Or you can try this...

★ Use diced lamb fillet instead of chicken.
★ Use mashed cannellini beans instead of chickpeas.
★ Warm and split some pita breads or use flatbreads instead of wraps.

Mexican scrambled eggs and bean wraps

Eating scrambled eggs for a late supper may help you to sleep more soundly. Eggs are a valuable source of vitamin D, which affects the neurons in your brain associated with sleep, as well as the essential amino acid tryptophan, a natural sedative.

SERVES 4
PREP: 10 minutes
COOK: 10 minutes

- 1 tbsp olive oil
- 1 bunch spring onions, thinly sliced
- 4 large multi-seed or multi-grain wraps
- 1 x 400 g/14 oz can refried beans
- 6 medium free-range eggs
- 4 tbsp chopped fresh coriander
- 1 ripe avocado, stoned, peeled and diced
- 60 g/2 oz grated Cheddar or Monterey Jack cheese
- 4 tbsp Greek yoghurt
- salt and freshly ground black pepper

Heat the oil in a non-stick pan set over a low heat. Add the spring onions and cook gently for 3–4 minutes.

Meanwhile, heat the wraps in a low oven or on a hot griddle pan.

Gently heat the refried beans in a pan set over a low heat.

Beat the eggs in a bowl and add the coriander plus some salt and pepper. Pour the mixture into the pan containing the spring onions and stir over a low heat until the eggs start to scramble and set. Take care not to over-cook them.

Spread the refried beans over the warmed wraps and top with the scrambled eggs. Sprinkle with the avocado and grated cheese and add a dollop of Greek yoghurt. Fold the tortillas over or roll them up and eat immediately.

Or you can try this ...

★ Substitute regular low-fat natural yoghurt or sour cream for the Greek yoghurt.
★ Instead of diced avocado, use guacamole.
★ Try stirring the grated cheese into the scrambled egg mixture.

Warm tabbouleh with tahini drizzle

SERVES 4
PREP: 15 minutes
COOK: 30 minutes

60 g/2 oz sultanas
200 g/7 oz bulgur wheat (dry weight)
240 ml/8 fl oz vegetable stock
1 red onion, finely chopped
1 bunch fresh flat-leaf parsley or mint, finely chopped
60 g/2 oz medjool dates, stoned and chopped
2 tbsp pumpkin and sunflower seeds
juice of 1 lemon
4 tbsp fruity green olive oil, plus extra for oiling
2 red or yellow peppers, deseeded and quartered
2 radicchio heads, cut into quarters lengthwise
60 g/2 oz hazelnuts or pistachios
200 g/7 oz soft goats' cheese, cut into pieces
salt and freshly ground black pepper

FOR THE TAHINI DRIZZLE:
2 tbsp tahini
1 tbsp lemon juice
2 tsp balsamic vinegar
1 tsp clear honey
1 garlic clove, crushed

The dried fruit, seeds and nuts add a plethora of sleep-friendly nutrients to the slightly nutty-tasting bulgur wheat, which contains high levels of magnesium, making it a great natural aid to sleep.

Put the sultanas in a bowl and pour some hot water over them. Leave to soak for at least 10 minutes until they plump up. Drain and set aside.

Put the bulgur wheat and stock in a saucepan and bring to the boil. Reduce the heat, cover the pan and simmer for 5 minutes. Remove from the heat and leave, covered, for at least another 5 minutes or until the grains of bulgur wheat are tender and have absorbed most or all of the stock. Transfer to a large bowl and mix in the drained sultanas, onion, herbs, dates, seeds, lemon juice and olive oil. Season to taste with salt and pepper.

While the tabbouleh is cooking, lightly oil a griddle pan and set over a medium to high heat. When it's hot, add the red or yellow peppers and cook for about 5 minutes until tender and starting to char around the edges.

Remove the peppers and set aside. Add the radicchio to the pan and cook for about 2 minutes until it starts to wilt and get slightly charred.

Place a dry frying pan over a medium heat and add the hazelnuts or pistachios. Toast for about 2 minutes, stirring frequently, until they start to turn golden brown – don't let them burn. Remove immediately.

Make the tahini drizzle: whisk all the ingredients together until smooth.

Divide the radicchio quarters between four serving plates and add the tabbouleh. Dot with the goats' cheese and sprinkle with the toasted nuts, peppers and tahini drizzle.

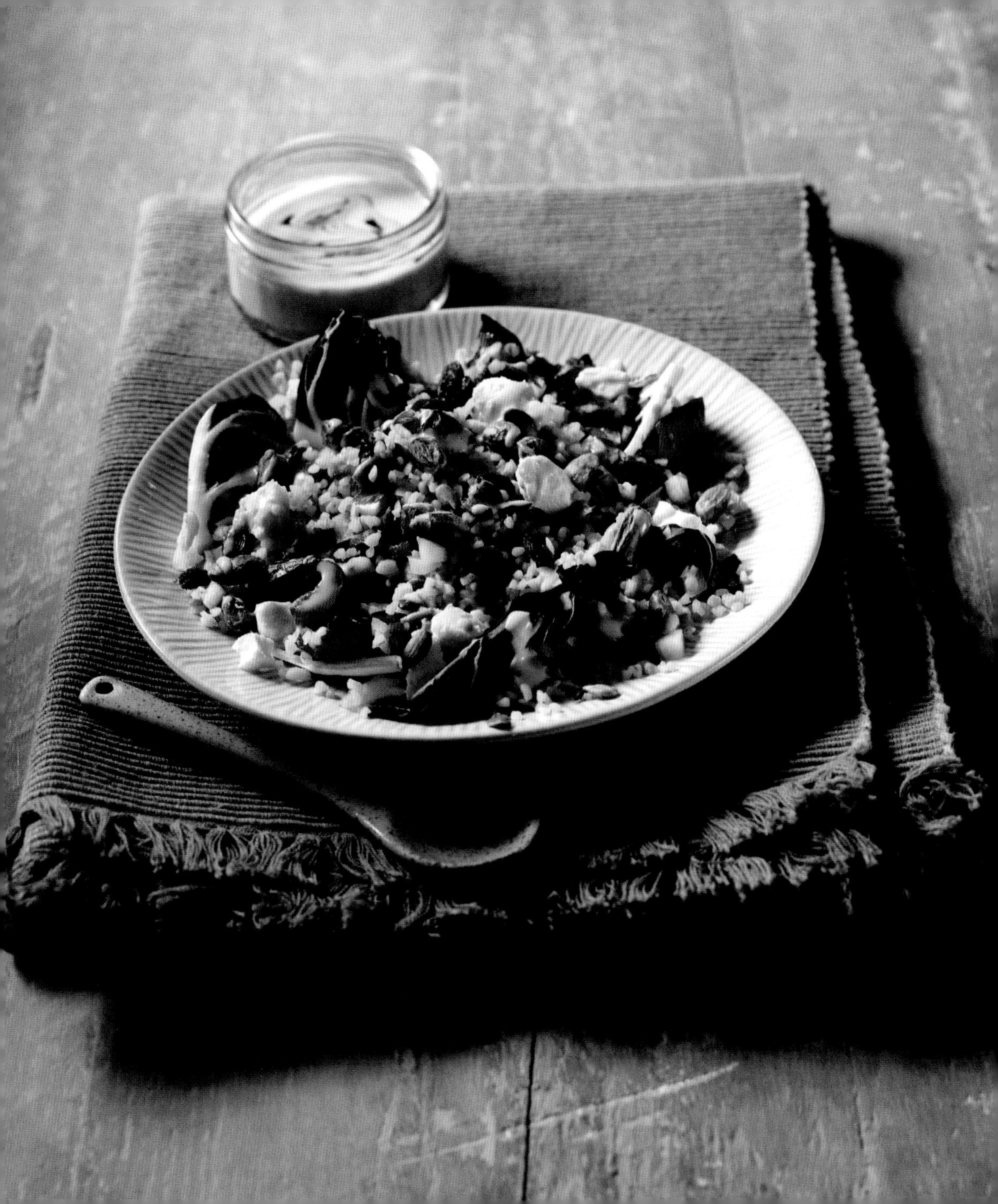

Warm lentil salad with smoked salmon rolls

SERVES 4
PREP: 10 minutes
COOK: 30 minutes

- 200 g/7 oz Puy or green lentils (dry weight)
- 3 tbsp olive oil, plus extra for drizzling
- 1 large onion, chopped
- 2 large carrots, diced
- 2 sticks celery, diced
- 3 garlic cloves, crushed
- grated zest and juice of 1 lemon
- 1 tbsp balsamic vinegar, plus extra for drizzling
- 1 bunch fresh flat-leaf parsley or dill, finely chopped
- 200 g/7 oz fine green beans, trimmed
- 150 g/5 oz thinly sliced smoked salmon
- salt and freshly ground black pepper
- Greek yoghurt and lemon wedges to serve

Lentils are one of the healthiest, most nutritious foods you can eat and they make a delicious and economical meal. They are high in protein and fibre as well as sleep-inducing vitamins and minerals.

Put the lentils in a saucepan and cover with cold water. Bring to the boil, then reduce the heat and simmer gently for about 20 minutes until they are tender but still retain a little 'bite'. Drain and refresh under cold water.

Meanwhile, heat the oil in a large frying pan set over a low heat. Add the onion, carrots, celery and garlic and cook gently, stirring occasionally, for about 10 minutes until soft and translucent.

Add the cooked lentils. Stir well and cook for 10 minutes, stirring occasionally. If the lentils start to stick, add a little stock or water. Stir in the lemon juice, balsamic vinegar and parsley or dill, and season to taste with salt and pepper. Remove from the heat and set aside to cool a little.

Cook the green beans in a pan of boiling water for 3–4 minutes. Refresh under cold running water and drain well.

When the lentils are lukewarm, divide them between four serving plates. Add the green beans and drizzle with olive oil and more balsamic vinegar. Roll up the smoked salmon slices and arrange on the side with a dollop of Greek yoghurt. Serve immediately with lemon wedges.

Or you can try this...

- ★ Omit the smoked salmon and sprinkle some grated Parmesan over the lentils before serving.
- ★ Add some diced cooked squash, sweet potato or pumpkin.

Tuscan stewed beans with pesto

Dark green leafy vegetables and beans provide a variety of sleep-inducing minerals. Use the freshest and best-quality vegetables you can find, preferably organic ones.

SERVES 4
PREP: 15 minutes
COOK: 1 hour

- 3 tbsp olive oil
- 1 large onion, chopped
- 1 leek, cleaned, trimmed and chopped
- 2 celery sticks, chopped
- 250 g/9 oz baby carrots (e.g. Chantenay), scrubbed and trimmed
- 2 garlic cloves, crushed
- 600 ml/1 pint vegetable stock
- 3 potatoes, peeled and cubed
- 3 fresh thyme sprigs, leaves stripped
- 2 fresh rosemary sprigs, leaves stripped and chopped
- 1 x 400 g/14 oz can borlotti or cannellini beans, drained and rinsed
- 250 g/9 oz curly kale or cavolo nero, ribs and stalks removed, leaves shredded
- 2–3 tbsp green pesto
- salt and freshly ground black pepper
- crusty wholemeal bread to serve

FOR THE PARMESAN CRISPS:

- 120 g/4 oz grated Parmesan cheese

Heat the olive oil in a large saucepan and cook the onion, leek, celery and carrots over a low heat for about 10 minutes, stirring occasionally, until softened but not coloured. Add the garlic and cook for 1 minute.

Add the stock and potatoes and bring to the boil. Reduce the heat and add the herbs. Simmer gently for 45 minutes or until all the vegetables are cooked and tender.

Stir in the beans and kale or cavolo nero and cook gently for 3–4 minutes – not too long or the leafy greens will lose their texture, colour and freshness. Stir in the pesto and season to taste with salt and pepper.

Meanwhile, make the Parmesan crisps. Preheat the oven to 180°C/350°F/gas mark 4 and line a non-stick baking sheet with baking parchment. Add four circular heaps of grated Parmesan and bake for 5 minutes or until the cheese melts and spreads. Remove from the oven and set aside to cool and crisp up.

Divide the stew between four wide shallow bowls and serve with the Parmesan crisps and crusty bread.

Or you can try this …

- ⭑ You can add any canned beans, e.g. flageolets, haricots or butterbeans.
- ⭑ Add a handful of macaroni or vermicelli about 10 minutes before the end of cooking.

Bubble and squeak cheesy omelette

SERVES 4
PREP: 15 minutes
COOK: 20 minutes

3 tbsp olive oil
1 red onion, thinly sliced
2 garlic cloves, crushed
200 g/7 oz leftover roast potatoes and/or parsnips, chopped
120 g/4 oz leftover cooked carrots and/or swede, chopped
120 g/4 oz leftover cooked cabbage and/or sprouts, shredded
6 medium free-range eggs
60 g/2 oz grated Cheddar or Parmesan cheese
salt and freshly ground black pepper

This is a great way to use up leftover roast, boiled or steamed vegetables, and everything is cooked in the same pan.

Heat the oil in a large wide frying pan set over a low to medium heat. Add the onion and garlic and cook, stirring occasionally, for about 5 minutes until tender and golden.

Add the potatoes and/or parsnips and cook, stirring, for 3–4 minutes until golden. Add the remaining vegetables and cook for 2–3 minutes.

Beat the eggs and season them lightly with salt and pepper. Pour into the pan and cook over a low heat for about 5 minutes until the omelette is set and golden brown underneath.

Preheat the grill to hot. Sprinkle the grated cheese over the top and pop the pan under the hot grill for 3 minutes or so until the omelette is set and golden brown on top and the cheese has melted.

Cut into wedges to serve. The omelette goes well with cold meat, chicken or ham.

Or you can try this...

★ Use leftover kale, spring greens, broccoli or spinach.
★ Add some frozen peas and chopped herbs.
★ Use cooked sweet potato, pumpkin or squash.

Tuna eggs Benedict

Eggs Benedict make a nutritious light supper when you're in a hurry. Tuna is a good source of vitamin B6, which is essential for making melatonin, while eggs contain tryptophan, which promotes sleep, especially when combined with carbohydrates.

SERVES 4
PREP: 10 minutes
COOK: 5 minutes

- 2 x 200 g/7 oz cans tuna in spring water, drained
- 4 tbsp light mayonnaise
- 1 tbsp white wine vinegar
- 4 medium free-range eggs
- 4 wholemeal English muffins
- 4 tbsp ready-made hollandaise sauce
- 1 small bunch chives, snipped
- salt and freshly ground black pepper

Mash the tuna lightly with a fork in a bowl and mix in the mayonnaise.

Heat some water in a wide shallow pan until it is just simmering. Add the vinegar and then carefully break the eggs, one at a time, into a small dish before sliding each one into the hot water. Leave them to poach in the gently simmering water for approximately 4 minutes until the whites are set but the yolks are still runny. If your pan isn't very big, you may have to cook the eggs in batches, or use an egg poacher if you have one.

Meanwhile, split the muffins and toast lightly on both sides. Spread with the mashed tuna.

Gently heat the hollandaise sauce in a small pan over a very low heat. Stir in the snipped chives.

Use a slotted spoon to remove the eggs from the pan and drain well. Pat dry with kitchen paper.

Place a poached egg on top of each tuna-topped muffin and drizzle the warm hollandaise sauce over the top. Season with a little salt and freshly ground black pepper and serve immediately.

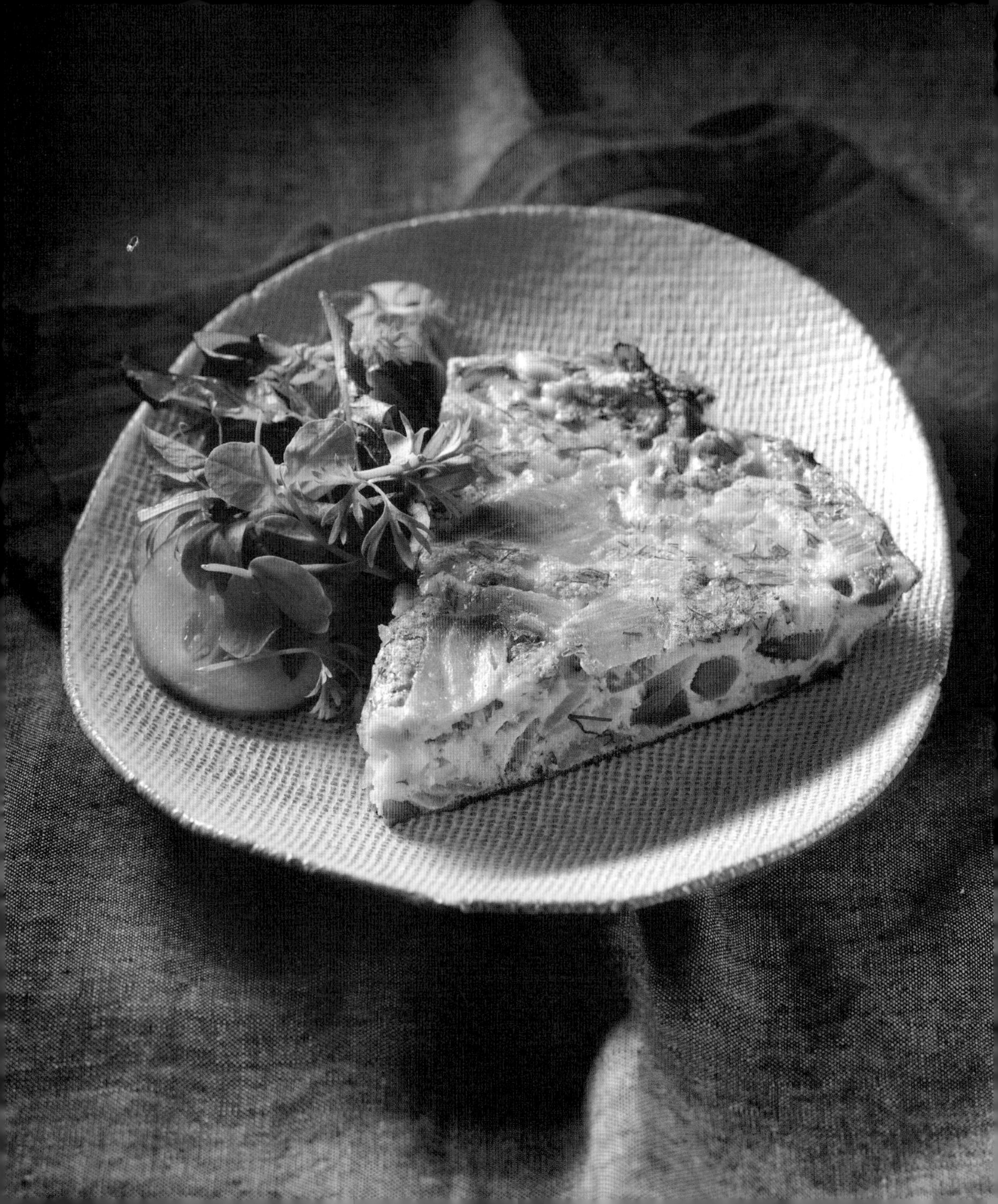

Smoked salmon frittata wedges

You don't have to use the best-quality smoked salmon to make this delicious frittata – smoked salmon trimmings are more economical and taste just as good.

SERVES 4
PREP: 10 minutes
COOK: 25–30 minutes

- 2 tbsp olive oil
- 1 onion, finely chopped
- 1 garlic clove, crushed
- 1 medium carrot, diced
- 2 celery sticks, diced
- 1 tbsp fennel seeds
- 1 tbsp cumin seeds
- 8 medium free-range eggs
- 1 small bunch fresh dill, chopped
- 200 g/7 oz smoked salmon, cut into small pieces
- salt and freshly ground black pepper
- salad to serve

Heat the oil in a large non-stick frying pan over a low to medium heat. Cook the onion, garlic, carrot and celery, stirring occasionally, for about 6–8 minutes until tender. Stir in the fennel and cumin seeds.

Beat the eggs in a clean bowl and stir in the dill, smoked salmon and a little salt and pepper.

Add the egg mixture to the hot pan and stir gently. Reduce the heat to barely simmering and cook gently for 10–15 minutes until the frittata is set and golden brown underneath and the top is just beginning to set.

Preheat your grill to hot. Pop the pan under the hot grill for a few minutes until the top is set and golden brown.

Slide the frittata out of the pan onto a serving plate or board. Set aside to cool slightly for a few minutes. Cut into four wedges and serve with some salad.

Or you can try this …

- For a veggie version, omit the smoked salmon and cook some diced squash, sweet potato or pumpkin with the onion and carrot.
- Substitute feathery fennel fronds, chives or tarragon for the dill.
- Add a handful of frozen peas or some diced courgettes.

Smoked salmon and sweet potato seedy fishcakes

SERVES 4
PREP: 20 minutes
CHILL: 30 minutes
COOK: 1–1¼ hours

- 600 g / 1 lb 5 oz sweet potatoes, washed
- 2 tbsp sunflower oil, plus extra for frying
- 1 bunch spring onions, finely chopped
- 1 tsp grated fresh root ginger
- 2 tsp black mustard seeds
- a pinch of ground cumin
- 1 small bunch fresh coriander, finely chopped
- 300 g / 10 oz hot smoked salmon fillet, skinned and flaked
- a few drops of soy sauce or teriyaki sauce
- 1–2 tbsp plain flour, plus extra for dusting
- salt and freshly ground black pepper
- Greek yoghurt and lime wedges to serve

You can make these fishcakes in advance and freeze them in batches before cooking them. Oily fish, such as salmon, are a good source of vitamin B6 which is essential for making melatonin.

Preheat the oven to 200°C/400°F/gas mark 6.

Pierce the sweet potatoes a few times with a fork or skewer and place them on a baking sheet. Bake in the preheated oven for 45–50 minutes, or until cooked and tender. Remove and set aside until they are cool enough to handle.

Meanwhile, heat the oil in a frying pan over a low heat and cook the spring onions and ginger for 5–8 minutes until softened but not browned. Add the mustard seeds and cook for 1 minute.

Scoop the flesh out of the sweet potato skins into a bowl, then stir in the spring onion mix, cumin, coriander, smoked salmon and soy or teriyaki sauce. Add enough flour to bind everything together. Season to taste with salt and pepper.

Divide the mixture into eight equal-sized portions and shape each one into a patty. Dust lightly with flour and chill, covered, in the fridge for at least 30 minutes to firm them up.

Heat a little sunflower oil in a large frying pan over a medium heat. When it's hot, add the fishcakes (you may need to do this in batches) and cook for 4–5 minutes each side until golden brown and crisp.

Serve the hot fishcakes immediately with some yoghurt and with lime wedges on the side for squeezing.

Chicken and cheese quesadillas with papaya salsa

Quesadillas are fun to make and infinitely versatile. Here they're served with a refreshing papaya salsa which is a good source of potassium.

SERVES 4
PREP: 20 minutes
COOK: 10–15 minutes

3 large red peppers
225 g/8 oz grated Cheddar cheese
4 large wholemeal tortillas
oil for brushing
2 skinned and boned cooked chicken breasts, shredded
½ red onion, diced
a handful of fresh coriander, chopped
salt and freshly ground black pepper

FOR THE PAPAYA SALSA:
1 large ripe papaya, skinned, deseeded and diced
½ red onion, finely diced
a handful of fresh coriander, finely chopped
juice of 1 lime

Preheat the grill on the highest setting. Place the peppers on a grill pan and pop under the hot grill for a few minutes, turning them occasionally, until they start to soften and the skin blisters and chars. Remove and place in a plastic bag.

When the peppers are cool enough to handle, peel off and discard the skins. Cut the peppers in half and remove the white ribs and seeds. Cut the flesh of two peppers into strips. Dice the flesh of the remaining pepper.

Make the salsa: put the diced red pepper in a bowl with the salsa ingredients and mix together. Season to taste.

Sprinkle the grated cheese over two tortillas, leaving a thin border around the edge. Place a tortilla in a lightly oiled non-stick frying pan set over a medium heat. When the cheese starts to melt, sprinkle on half of the red pepper strips, the chicken and red onion and a little coriander. Season lightly with salt and pepper.

Place a tortilla on top to cover and enclose the filling, pressing lightly around the edges. Cook for 1–2 minutes until golden underneath. Using a slice, carefully turn the quesadilla over to cook the other side for 1–2 minutes.

Remove from the pan and keep warm while you assemble and cook the remaining quesadilla in the same way.

Cut each quesadilla into wedges and serve immediately with the salsa.

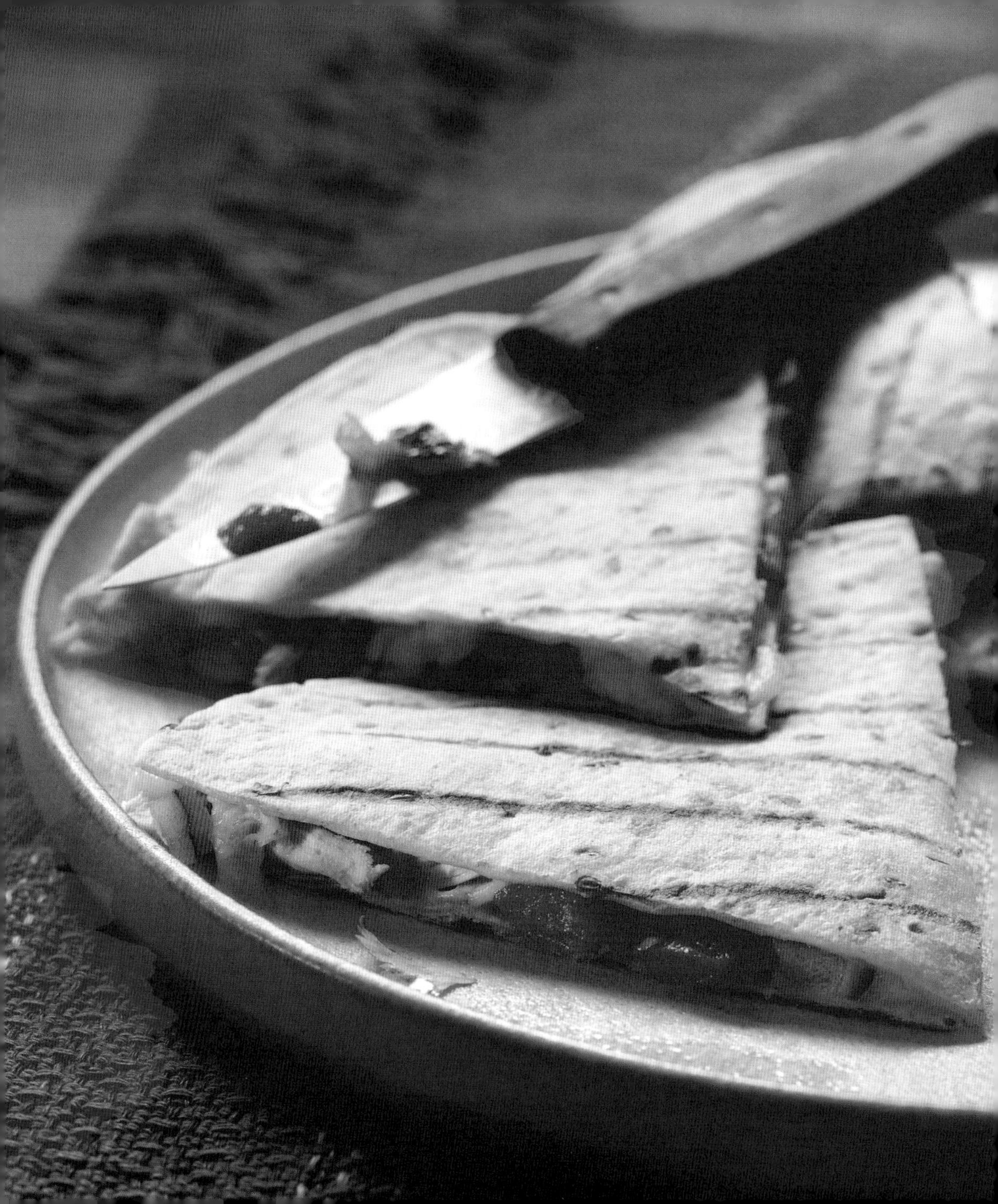

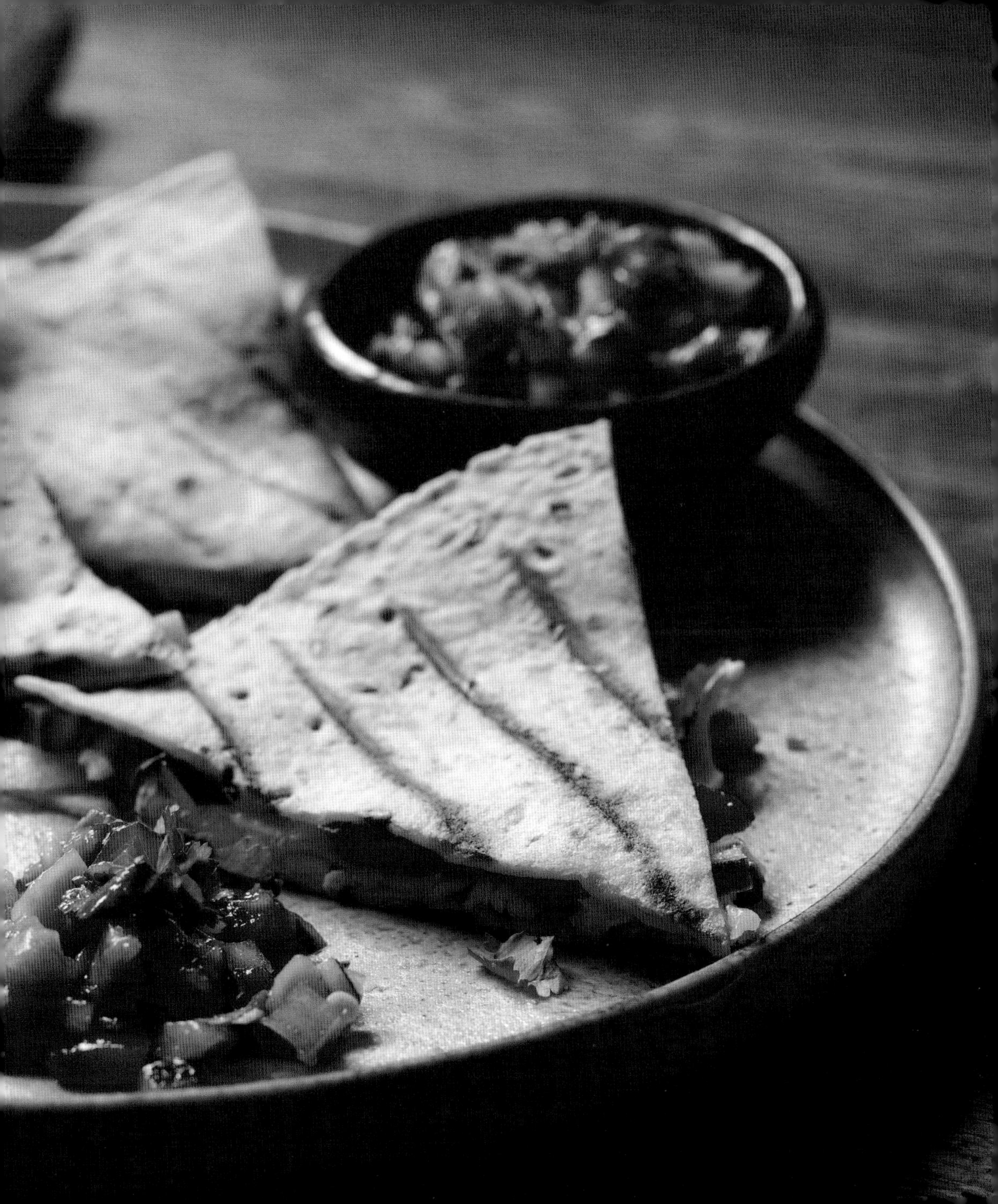

Savoury porridge with spinach and mushrooms

SERVES 4
PREP: 10 minutes
COOK: 30 minutes

- 3 tbsp olive oil
- 15 g/½ oz unsalted butter
- 1 onion, diced
- 1 garlic clove, crushed
- 400 g/14 oz mushrooms, sliced
- 3 fresh thyme sprigs, leaves stripped
- 150 g/5 oz oats, e.g. pinhead
- 900 ml/1½ pints vegetable stock
- 200 g/7 oz baby spinach leaves
- 120 g/4 oz grated Gruyère or Cheddar cheese
- salt and freshly ground black pepper

If you've always eaten porridge with honey or sugar and cream, it's time to think again and try an equally soothing savoury version. Oats are not only low GI, helping to regulate your blood sugar levels, but also high in magnesium.

Heat the olive oil and butter in a non-stick saucepan set over a low heat. Add the onion and garlic and cook for 5 minutes, stirring occasionally, until softened. Stir in the mushrooms and cook gently, stirring once or twice, until tender and golden.

Stir in the thyme leaves and oatmeal and, after 1–2 minutes, add the stock. Increase the heat a little and simmer gently, stirring occasionally, for about 15 minutes or until the oats have absorbed the stock and you have a moist porridge – it shouldn't be too dry. You're looking for the consistency of a slightly wet and soupy risotto.

Stir in the spinach leaves and leave for 1 minute until they turn bright green and wilt into the porridge. Stir in most of the grated cheese and season to taste with salt and pepper.

Ladle the porridge into four shallow serving bowls and sprinkle the remaining cheese over the top. Eat immediately.

Or you can try this…

- ★ Top with some crisp rashers of bacon or a fried egg.
- ★ Use dried porcini mushrooms and add the soaking liquid to the stock.
- ★ Add a handful of chopped fresh herbs, whichever ones you fancy or have to hand.

Butterbean and sweet potato soup

This autumnal soup can be served as a light supper with some crusty bread.

SERVES 4
PREP: 15 minutes
COOK: 45 minutes

2 tbsp olive oil
1 large onion, finely chopped
2 garlic cloves, crushed
a pinch of caster sugar
900 g/2 lb sweet potatoes, peeled and cubed
1 tsp ground cumin
1 tsp smoked paprika
1.2 litres/2 pints hot vegetable stock
1 x 400 g/14 oz can butterbeans, drained and rinsed
120 ml/4 fl oz crème fraîche
salt and freshly ground black pepper
60 g/2 oz plain tortilla chips, coarsely crushed
6 0g/2 oz grated Cheddar cheese

Heat the oil in a large saucepan and cook the onion and garlic over a low heat, stirring occasionally, for about 10 minutes until tender but not coloured. Stir in the sugar and add the sweet potatoes. Cook gently, stirring occasionally, for 5 minutes until golden. Add the spices and cook for 1 minute.

Add the hot stock and bring to the boil. Reduce the heat, cover the pan and simmer gently for 20 minutes until the sweet potatoes are tender. Add most of the beans, reserving a few for garnishing, and heat through for a couple of minutes.

Blitz the soup to a smooth purée in a blender or food processor, or use a stick blender. Season to taste with salt and pepper, and return to the pan. Stir in the crème fraîche and reheat gently.

Ladle the hot soup into four shallow bowls. Sprinkle with the reserved beans, tortilla chips and grated cheese and serve immediately.

Or you can try this…

- ★ Use butternut squash, pumpkin or even parsnips, swede and carrots, instead of sweet potatoes.
- ★ Any grated hard cheese works well – try Emmenthal, Gruyère or Parmesan.

Classic chicken soup

SERVES 6–8
PREP: 15 minutes
COOK: 2¼–2½ hours

1 x 1.5 kg/3 lb oven-ready chicken
1 large onion, diced
3 carrots, diced
2 leeks, cleaned, trimmed and shredded
4 celery sticks, diced
2 garlic cloves, crushed
2 bay leaves
3 fresh thyme sprigs
1.8 litres/3 pints water
225 g/8 oz vermicelli noodles
juice of ½ lemon (optional)
1 large bunch fresh flat-leaf parsley, finely chopped
sea salt and freshly ground black pepper

Soothing and filling on a cold day, this is comfort food at its very best. All the goodness from the chicken is absorbed into the delicious broth. Chicken soup is a great way to get vitamin B6 which is essential for the production of melatonin.

Place the chicken in a large heavy-based saucepan. Add the onion, carrots, leeks, celery, garlic, bay leaves and thyme. Pour in the water and add some salt and a good grinding of black pepper.

Set the pan over a high heat and bring to the boil, skimming off any dark coloured scum on the surface.

Reduce the heat to a simmer and partially cover the pan with a lid. Cook very gently for about 2 hours until the vegetables are tender and the chicken is thoroughly cooked and starting to fall off the bones.

Remove the chicken from the pan and set aside until it's cool enough to handle. Discard the skin and remove the meat from the carcass. Cut the meat into pieces and return it to the soup together with the vermicelli and most of the parsley.

Simmer for about 10 minutes until the vermicelli is cooked and tender. Fish out the bay leaves and check the seasoning, adding more salt and pepper if required. If wished, stir in the lemon juice.

Ladle the soup into bowls and sprinkle with the remaining parsley.

Or you can try this...

★ Add a chicken bouillon cube or powder to the water for extra flavour.
★ Cut the vegetables into larger pieces.
★ Instead of pasta or noodles, add some cubed potatoes.

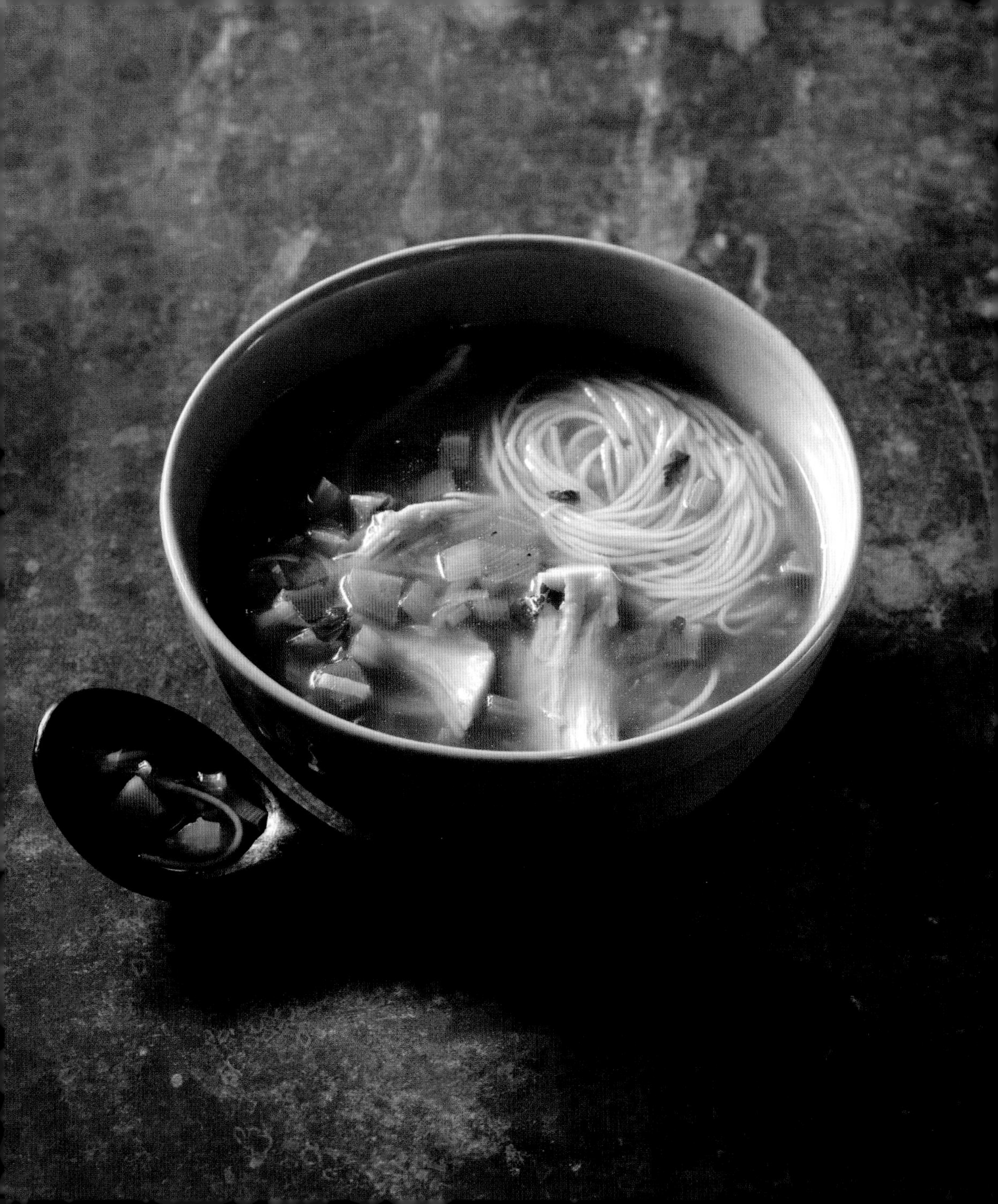

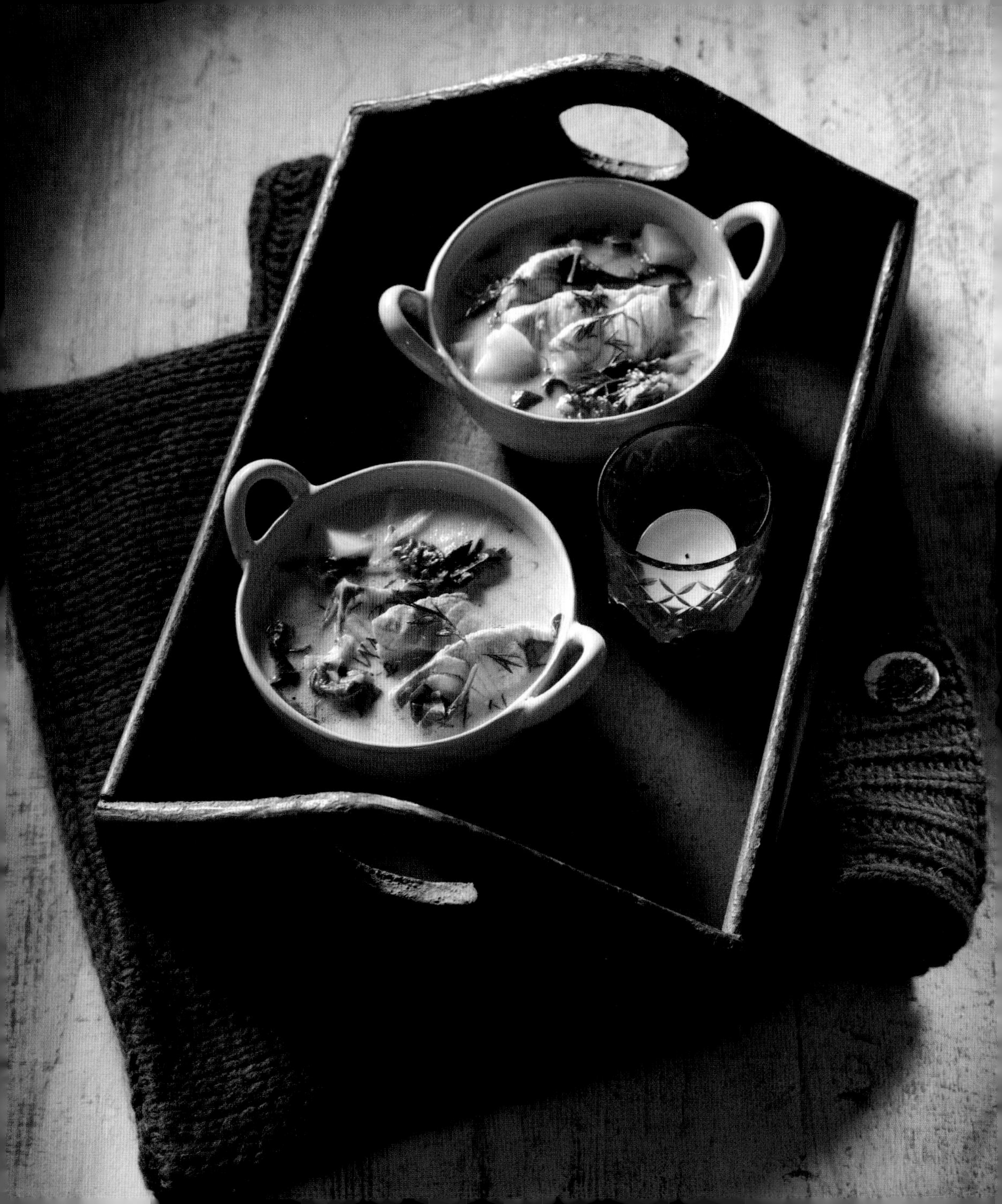

Swedish salmon, potato and dill soup

The quality of the salmon will affect the flavour of this 'meal in a bowl', so try to source wild salmon which is better nutritionally. Salmon contains sleep-enhancing magnesium, vitamins B6 and D, and tryptophan. Potatoes and spinach promote good digestion.

SERVES 4
PREP: 15 minutes
COOK: 25 minutes

30 g/1 oz butter
1 large onion, chopped
2 leeks, cleaned, trimmed and shredded
1 kg/2 lb 4 oz waxy potatoes, peeled and cubed
900 ml/1½ pints fish stock
2 bay leaves
2 ripe tomatoes, chopped
400 g/14 oz salmon fillet, skinned, boned and thickly sliced
200 g/7 oz baby spinach leaves
120 ml/4 fl oz soured cream or crème fraîche
1 small bunch fresh dill, chopped, plus a few sprigs to garnish
salt and freshly ground black pepper

Melt the butter in a large saucepan and cook the onion and leeks over a low to medium heat, stirring occasionally, until softened but not coloured. Add the potatoes and cook, stirring, for 6–8 minutes.

Add the fish stock and bay leaves and bring to the boil. Reduce the heat and add the tomatoes. Simmer gently, partially covered, for 10 minutes until the potatoes are cooked and tender.

Add the salmon and spinach and continue cooking gently for 5 minutes until the salmon is cooked through but not flaking. Season to taste with salt and pepper, then gently stir in the soured cream or crème fraîche and dill.

Ladle the soup into shallow bowls and garnish with dill sprigs. Serve immediately.

Or you can try this …

★ Add some sliced or diced carrots and swede.
★ Stir in some more chopped tomatoes or use canned.
★ Instead of spinach, use shredded kale or spring greens.

Cauliflower cheese jackets

SERVES 4
PREP: 10 minutes
COOK: 1 hour

- 4 large sweet potatoes or regular potatoes
- 400 g/14 oz cauliflower florets
- 1 tbsp whole grain mustard
- 200 g/7 oz low-fat natural yoghurt
- a handful of fresh parsley, finely chopped
- 200 g/7 oz grated Cheddar cheese
- salt and freshly ground black pepper

If you've never thought of stuffing a baked sweet potato or regular baking potato with cauliflower cheese, now's the time to try it. It will both fill you up and provide vitamin B6 and potassium to help you sleep better.

Preheat the oven to 200°C/400°F/gas mark 6.

Scrub the sweet potatoes (or potatoes) under running water and pat dry with kitchen paper. Prick them all over with a fork and place on a baking sheet. Bake in the preheated oven for 50–60 minutes until they yield slightly when you press them gently. Alternatively, you can microwave them for about 8 minutes until tender.

Meanwhile, cook the cauliflower in a pan of lightly salted boiling water for about 5 minutes until just tender (not mushy). Drain well and cut into smaller pieces.

Cut a cross in the top of each sweet potato (or potato) and press gently on the sides to open them up. Scoop out the inside and mash with the mustard, yoghurt, parsley and half the cheese. Mix in the cauliflower and season to taste.

Stuff the potato and cauliflower mixture back into the skins and arrange on a baking sheet. Sprinkle the remaining cheese over the top and pop back into the oven for 10 minutes until golden brown and bubbling.

Or you can try this…

- ★ Substitute broccoli florets for cauliflower.
- ★ Sprinkle with a pinch of paprika or cayenne pepper.
- ★ Use coarsely grated Parmesan or Gruyère instead of Cheddar cheese.

Sweet potato 'sliders'

Using roasted, baked or griddled sliced vegetables instead of burger buns is both delicious and healthy. Sweet potatoes are ideal for this and provide potassium, which aids good digestion, relaxes nerves and muscles, and can prevent night cramps.

SERVES 4
PREP: 20 minutes
CHILL: 15–30 minutes
COOK: 20–25 minutes

500 g/1 lb 2 oz minced chicken
1 red onion, diced
3 garlic cloves, crushed
1 tsp grated fresh root ginger
1 stalk lemongrass, peeled and finely sliced
grated zest and juice of 1 lime
1 small bunch fresh coriander
flour for dusting
2 medium sweet potatoes, scrubbed
olive oil for brushing
1 tsp smoked paprika
4 tbsp 0% fat Greek yoghurt
¼ small cucumber, diced
salt and freshly ground black pepper
salad to serve

Preheat the oven to 180°C/350°F/gas mark 4.

Pulse the chicken, onion, 2 garlic cloves, ginger, lemongrass, lime zest and coriander in a food processor until well combined. Season lightly with salt and pepper.

With lightly floured hands, divide the mixture into four equal-sized portions and shape into burgers. Cover and chill in the fridge for 15–30 minutes to firm them up.

Cut the sweet potatoes into eight 2.5 cm (1 in) thick rounds. Brush each one lightly with olive oil and place on a baking sheet. Dust with paprika and sprinkle with salt and pepper. Bake in the preheated oven for 20–25 minutes, turning them over after 10 minutes, until just tender and golden brown.

Meanwhile, cook the burgers in a lightly oiled griddle pan or under a preheated hot grill for about 8 minutes on each side, until cooked right through and golden brown.

Mix together the yoghurt, lime juice, cucumber and the remaining garlic clove. Season to taste.

Assemble the sliders: place a baked sweet potato slice on each serving plate and top with a chicken burger and a spoonful of the yoghurt mixture. Cover with another sweet potato slice and serve immediately with some salad.

2

FILLING SUPPERS

Baked chicken and broccoli gratin

SERVES 4
PREP: 15 minutes
COOK: 35–45 minutes

2 tbsp olive oil
1 onion, finely chopped
450 g/1 lb skinned chicken breast fillets, cut into chunks
400 g/14 oz broccoli, cut into florets
60 g/2 oz fresh white breadcrumbs
4 tbsp grated Cheddar cheese
cayenne pepper for dusting

FOR THE CHEESE SAUCE:
60 g/2 oz butter
60 g/2 oz plain flour
480 ml/16 fl oz milk
100 g/3½ oz grated Cheddar cheese
salt and freshly ground black pepper

This homely supper is surprisingly filling. The broccoli, cheese and milk all provide calcium, which helps our brain make use of sleep-enhancing tryptophan.

Preheat the oven to 200°C/400°F/gas mark 6.

Heat the oil in a frying pan set over a medium heat. Add the onion and cook for 5 minutes, stirring occasionally. Stir in the chicken and cook for about 5 minutes, turning a few times, until lightly browned all over. Remove from the pan and transfer to an ovenproof baking dish.

Meanwhile, steam the broccoli over a pan of simmering water for 4–5 minutes until just tender. Drain well and add to the baking dish.

Make the cheese sauce: melt the butter in a non-stick pan over a low heat and stir in the flour with a wooden spoon. Cook for 2 minutes until it smells 'biscuity' and then add the milk, a little at a time, stirring or whisking until smooth. Keep stirring over a low heat until the sauce thickens. Remove the pan from the heat and stir in the cheese, then season to taste.

Pour the cheese sauce over the chicken and broccoli, then sprinkle the breadcrumbs and Cheddar over the top.

Bake in the preheated oven for 20–30 minutes until bubbling and golden brown on top. Dust with cayenne and serve immediately.

Or you can try this...

★ Use purple-sprouting or tenderstem broccoli.
★ Add a few cauliflower florets.
★ Use grated Parmesan, Gruyère or Lancashire cheese in the sauce.

Chicken risotto with cavolo nero

Risotto is very soothing at the end of a long day. It's cooked in one pan and can be eaten in a bowl as a TV supper so there's minimal fuss and washing up.

SERVES 4
PREP: 10 minutes
COOK: 25–30 minutes

2 tbsp olive oil
15 g/½ oz butter
1 onion, diced
2 leeks, trimmed, cleaned and thinly sliced
300 g/10 oz Arborio or Carnaroli risotto rice
1.2 litres/2 pints hot chicken stock
300 g/10 oz cavolo nero cabbage (or kale), shredded
450 g/1 lb cooked chicken (skinned and boned), shredded
juice of ½ lemon
a few sprigs of fresh basil, chopped
60 g/2 oz grated Parmesan
salt and freshly ground black pepper

Heat the olive oil and butter in a large saucepan and cook the onion and leeks over a low heat, stirring occasionally, for about 6–8 minutes until tender but not coloured.

Add the rice and cook for 1–2 minutes, stirring, until it starts to crackle and all the grains are glistening and coated with oil and butter.

Start adding the hot stock, a ladleful at a time, stirring with each addition until the liquid has been absorbed.

When most of the stock has been added and the rice is tender, gently stir in the cavolo nero with the last ladleful of stock. Simmer gently, stirring, until the liquid has been absorbed and the rice is just tender but not mushy.

Stir in the chicken, lemon juice and basil and warm through very gently. Check the seasoning, adding salt and pepper to taste.

Take the pan off the heat and stir in the Parmesan. Rest for 5 minutes before serving.

Or you can try this…

★ Top the risotto with some roasted fennel, shallots or spring onions.
★ Add podded fresh peas, broad beans, sugar snap peas and baby spinach.
★ Stir in some pesto at the end and sprinkle with pine nuts.

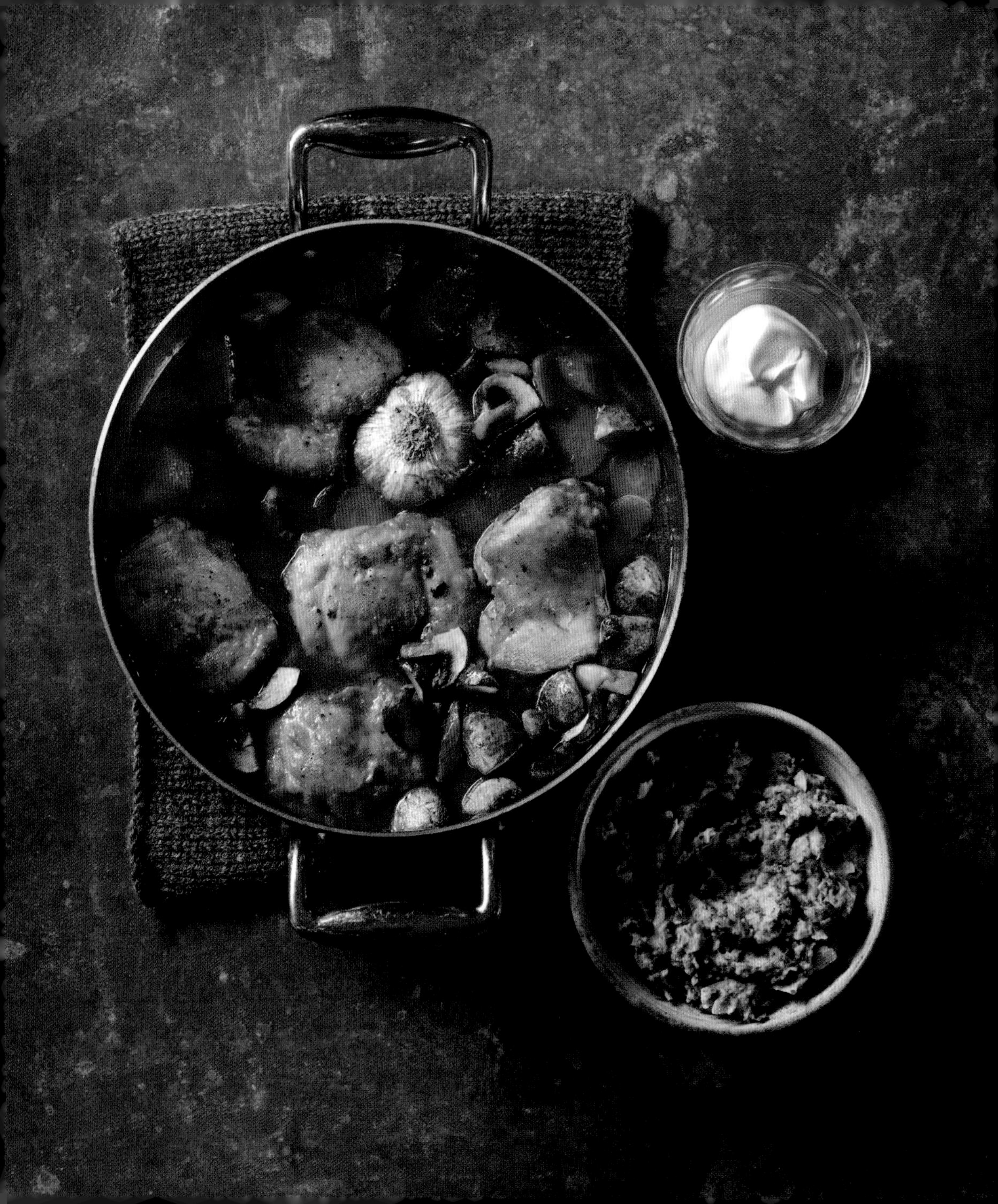

Hunter's chicken with smashed white beans

The smashed beans help to soak up the delicious sauce, as well as providing protein and dietary fibre. Both the butterbeans and spinach provide calcium, magnesium and potassium.

SERVES 4
PREP: 15 minutes
COOK: 1 hour

8 chicken thighs, skinned
2 tbsp flour
2 tbsp olive oil
15 g/½ oz (1 tbsp) butter
1 garlic bulb, unpeeled and cut in half horizontally
2 carrots, chopped
350 g/12 oz mushrooms, halved or quartered
a few sprigs of fresh rosemary
420 ml/14 fl oz chicken stock
60 ml/2 fl oz crème fraîche.
salt and freshly ground black pepper

FOR THE WHITE BEANS:
3 tbsp olive oil
1 onion, finely chopped
1 fresh rosemary sprig
200 g/7 oz baby spinach leaves
2 x 400 g/14 oz cans butterbeans, drained and rinsed
grated zest of 1 lemon
salt and freshly ground black pepper

Dust the chicken lightly with flour. Heat the oil and butter in a large heavy saucepan set over a medium heat. Add the chicken thighs and cook, turning them occasionally, until they are golden brown on all sides.

Add the garlic, carrots and mushrooms and cook for 5 minutes, then add the rosemary and chicken stock. Cover and simmer gently for about 45 minutes until the chicken is cooked through and really tender and the sauce has reduced. Season to taste with salt and pepper, and squeeze the garlic out of its skin into the sauce. Stir in the crème fraîche.

While the chicken is cooking, make the white beans. Heat the olive oil in a small pan and cook the onion and rosemary gently for about 10 minutes until really tender. Add the spinach and cook for 1–2 minutes until it wilts. Remove the rosemary and blitz the onion and spinach with the beans and lemon zest in a blender or food processor until you have a thick purée. Reheat in the pan and season to taste.

Spoon the chicken in its sauce onto four serving plates and serve with the beans.

Or you can try this...

★ Use chicken joints, including breasts and wings.
★ Serve with brown rice instead of smashed beans.
★ Use canned cannellini or haricot beans.

Cool turkey fajitas with guacamole

SERVES 4
PREP: 10 minutes
COOK: 20 minutes

olive oil for brushing
2 large red onions, thinly sliced
2 red, green or yellow peppers, deseeded and sliced
a handful of fresh coriander, chopped
600 g / 1 lb 5 oz turkey breast, skinned and cut into strips
8 wholemeal tortillas
salt and freshly ground black pepper
soured cream to serve

FOR THE GUACAMOLE:
½ red onion, diced
1 garlic clove, crushed
½ tsp sea salt crystals
2 ripe avocados, stoned, peeled and coarsely mashed
juice of 1 lime
1 small bunch fresh coriander, chopped
freshly ground black pepper

These cool fajitas and the accompanying guacamole are made without chillies or hot salsa. Scientists think that hot spicy foods can interfere with our ability to sleep by irritating the upper digestive tract and causing heartburn and restlessness.

Make the guacamole: crush the red onion, garlic and salt using a pestle and mortar. Mix with the avocado, lime juice and coriander. Add a grinding of black pepper and set aside.

Lightly brush a non-stick ridged griddle pan with oil and place over a medium heat. Add the red onions and peppers and cook for 8–10 minutes, turning occasionally, until softened, slightly charred and the onions are starting to caramelize. Remove from the pan, stir in the coriander and some salt and pepper, and keep warm.

Increase the heat and add the turkey to the pan. Cook for 5–8 minutes, turning occasionally, until the turkey is cooked right through and golden brown. Remove from the pan.

Put the tortillas in the hot pan – just long enough to warm them through. Or you can warm them in the microwave or wrapped in foil in a low oven.

Pile some turkey and griddled vegetables onto each tortilla. Top with the guacamole and soured cream, then fold over or roll up.

Or you can try this…

- Use chicken instead of turkey. For speed, buy packs of turkey or chicken cut into strips for stir-frying.
- Make some seafood fajitas with grilled prawns.

Cheesy pork steaks with stir-fried spring greens

Pork is an excellent source of vitamin B6 and potassium, while the cheese contains naturally sedating tryptophan. Serve this dish with some healthy carbs, such as wholegrain bread or brown rice, which will promote the absorption of tryptophan into the bloodstream.

SERVES 4
PREP: 15 minutes
COOK: 20 minutes

- 3 tbsp olive oil, plus extra for brushing
- 1 large onion, thinly sliced
- 120 g/4 oz grated Cheddar cheese
- 2 tsp Dijon mustard
- 90 ml/3 fl oz half-fat crème fraîche
- 4 lean pork loin steaks

FOR THE STIR-FRIED SPRING GREENS:

- 1 tsp mustard seeds
- 1 small bunch spring onions, thinly sliced
- 1 garlic clove, crushed
- 1 tsp grated fresh root ginger
- 450 g/1 lb spring greens, shredded
- salt and freshly ground black pepper

Heat two tablespoons of the oil in a frying pan set over a low to medium heat. Add the onion and cook for 6–8 minutes, stirring occasionally, until really tender.

Transfer the onion to a bowl and mix with the grated cheese, mustard and crème fraîche.

Preheat the grill. Brush the pork steaks lightly with oil on both sides and place them in a foil-lined grill pan. Cook under the hot grill for 3–4 minutes on each side.

Spoon the cheesy onion mixture on top of the pork and pop back under the grill for 2–3 minutes until the pork is cooked through and the topping is golden and bubbling.

Meanwhile, heat the remaining oil in a non-stick frying pan set over a high heat. Add the mustard seeds to the hot pan and cook for 1 minute until they start to pop. Reduce the heat and add the spring onions, garlic and ginger. Cook for 2 minutes and then stir in the spring greens. Stir-fry for 3–5 minutes until just tender but still a little crisp. Season to taste.

Serve the cheesy pork steaks immediately with the stir-fried spring greens.

Pork ragù with creamy mushrooms and fettuccine

SERVES 4
PREP: 10 minutes
SOAK: 30 minutes
COOK: 30 minutes

15 g/½oz dried porcini mushrooms
500 g/1 lb 2 oz pork fillet (tenderloin), all visible fat removed and cut into thin strips
3 tbsp olive oil
1 onion, thinly sliced
450 g/1 lb mushrooms, e.g. chestnut, morels and ceps, sliced
300 ml/½ pint chicken stock
200 ml/7 fl oz half-fat crème fraîche
grated zest of 1 lemon
500 g/1 lb 2 oz fettuccine (dried weight)
salt and freshly ground black pepper
a handful of fresh parsley, chopped

All edible mushrooms contain nutrients, including vitamin D and potassium. The dried porcini give this pasta dish its distinctive flavour. If you can get hold of wild mushrooms, use them in preference to cultivated ones.

Put the porcini in a heatproof jug or bowl and pour over some boiling water. Set aside to soak for at least 30 minutes. Drain well, straining and reserving the soaking liquid.

Season the pork with salt and pepper. Heat the oil in a wide deep sauté pan set over a medium to high heat and cook the pork, turning it occasionally, for about 5 minutes until browned all over. Set aside.

Add the onion and sliced mushrooms to the pan and cook, stirring occasionally, until the mushrooms are golden and the onions have softened but not coloured.

Return the pork to the pan together with the drained porcini. Stir into the onion and mushrooms, then add the chicken stock and the reserved porcini soaking liquid.

Simmer for 10–15 minutes until the pork is cooked and tender and the liquid has reduced. Stir in the crème fraîche and lemon zest and heat through gently for 2–3 minutes. Check the seasoning.

Meanwhile, cook the pasta in a large pan of lightly salted boiling water according to the instructions on the packet. Drain well.

Divide the cooked pasta between four serving plates and top with the pork ragù. Sprinkle with parsley and serve.

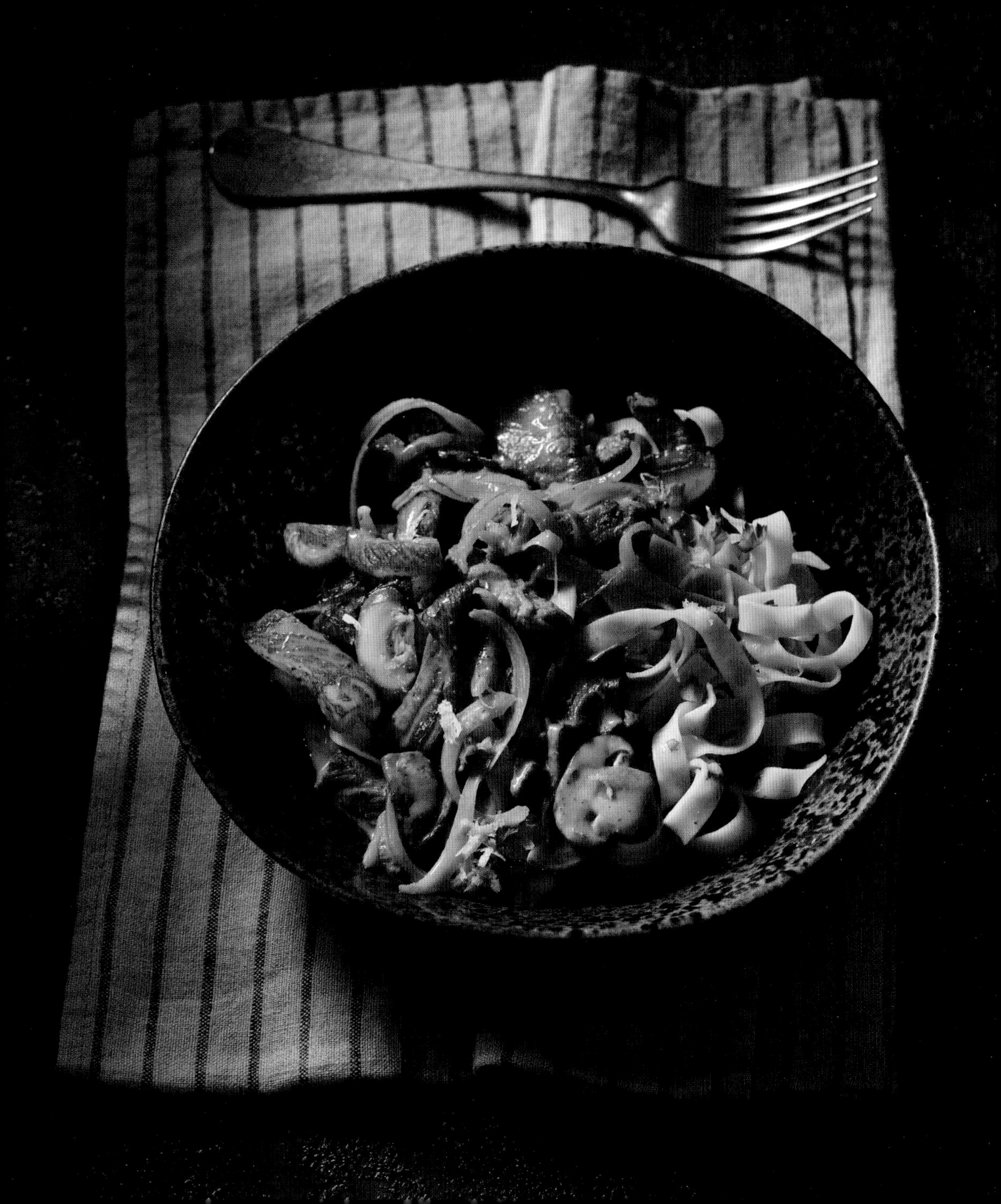

Creamy salmon and dill potato bake

SERVES 4
PREP: 15 minutes
COOK: 50–60 minutes

500 g/1 lb 2 oz potatoes
400 g/14 oz baby spinach leaves
500 g/1 lb 2 oz skinned salmon fillets, cut into chunks
15 g/½ oz butter, diced
green vegetables to serve

FOR THE WHITE SAUCE:
60 g/2 oz butter
60 g/2 oz plain flour
480 ml/16 fl oz milk
a pinch of ground nutmeg
grated zest of 1 lemon
a handful of fresh dill, chopped
salt and freshly ground black pepper

This delicious bake doesn't take long to assemble. Just pop it in the oven and relax while it cooks to an appetizing golden brown. Salmon is a good way to get some vitamin D into your diet.

Peel the potatoes and cook them whole in a pan of boiling salted water for 10–12 minutes. Drain and set aside to cool.

Preheat the oven to 200°C/400°F/gas mark 6.

Put the spinach in a colander and pour some boiling water over it. Drain well, squeezing out the excess water. Transfer to an ovenproof baking dish with the salmon.

Make the white sauce: melt the butter in a non-stick pan set over a low heat and stir in the flour with a wooden spoon. Cook for 2 minutes until it smells 'biscuity' and then add the milk, a little at a time, stirring or whisking until smooth. Keep stirring over a low heat until the sauce thickens. Remove from the heat and season with the nutmeg, lemon zest, dill and some salt and pepper.

Pour the white sauce over the salmon and spinach. Slice the potatoes thinly and arrange on top in overlapping slices to completely cover the salmon and spinach. Dot the top with butter.

Bake in the preheated oven for 30–40 minutes until the salmon is cooked through and the potatoes are golden brown and crisp. Serve immediately with green vegetables.

Lentil and roots cottage pie

This veggie cottage pie is perfect for supper on a cold day. The combination of mushrooms, spinach, sweet potatoes and cheese provide a jackpot of sleep-enhancing nutrients.

SERVES 4
PREP: 20 minutes
COOK: 55–60 minutes

3 tbsp olive oil
1 onion, chopped
1 leek, washed, trimmed and sliced
2 garlic cloves, crushed
2 carrots, diced
400 g/14 oz mushrooms, quartered
200 g/7 oz canned or fresh chopped tomatoes
300 ml/½ pint vegetable stock
1 x 400 g/14 oz can green lentils, drained and rinsed
400 g/14 oz baby spinach leaves
1 tbsp balsamic vinegar

FOR THE TOPPING:
900 g/2 lb mixed root vegetables, peeled and cubed, e.g. sweet potatoes with swede, parsnips or potatoes
3 tbsp milk
3 tbsp olive oil or butter
salt and freshly ground black pepper
60 g/2 oz grated Cheddar cheese

Preheat the oven to 200°C/400°F/gas mark 6.

Heat the oil in a saucepan set over a low heat. Add the onion, leek, garlic and carrots and cook, stirring occasionally, for 8–10 minutes until tender. Add the mushrooms and cook for 5 minutes.

Add the tomatoes and stock and bring to the boil. Reduce the heat, stir in the lentils and simmer gently for 15–20 minutes until the sauce reduces and thickens and the vegetables are cooked. Stir in the spinach and cook for 1 minute until it wilts. Season to taste with salt and pepper and a few drops of balsamic vinegar.

Meanwhile, cook the root vegetables for the topping in a pan of boiling water until tender. Drain well and mash coarsely with the milk and oil or butter. Season with salt and pepper.

Spoon the lentil and vegetable mixture into an ovenproof dish and cover with the mashed roots right up to the edges. Sprinkle the cheese over the top and bake in the preheated oven for 25–30 minutes until the edges are bubbling and the top is crisp and golden brown. Serve immediately.

Or you can try this...

- ★ Use canned beans instead of lentils.
- ★ Flavour the filling or even the root vegetable topping with some chopped herbs, e.g. parsley, thyme, oregano or bay leaves.

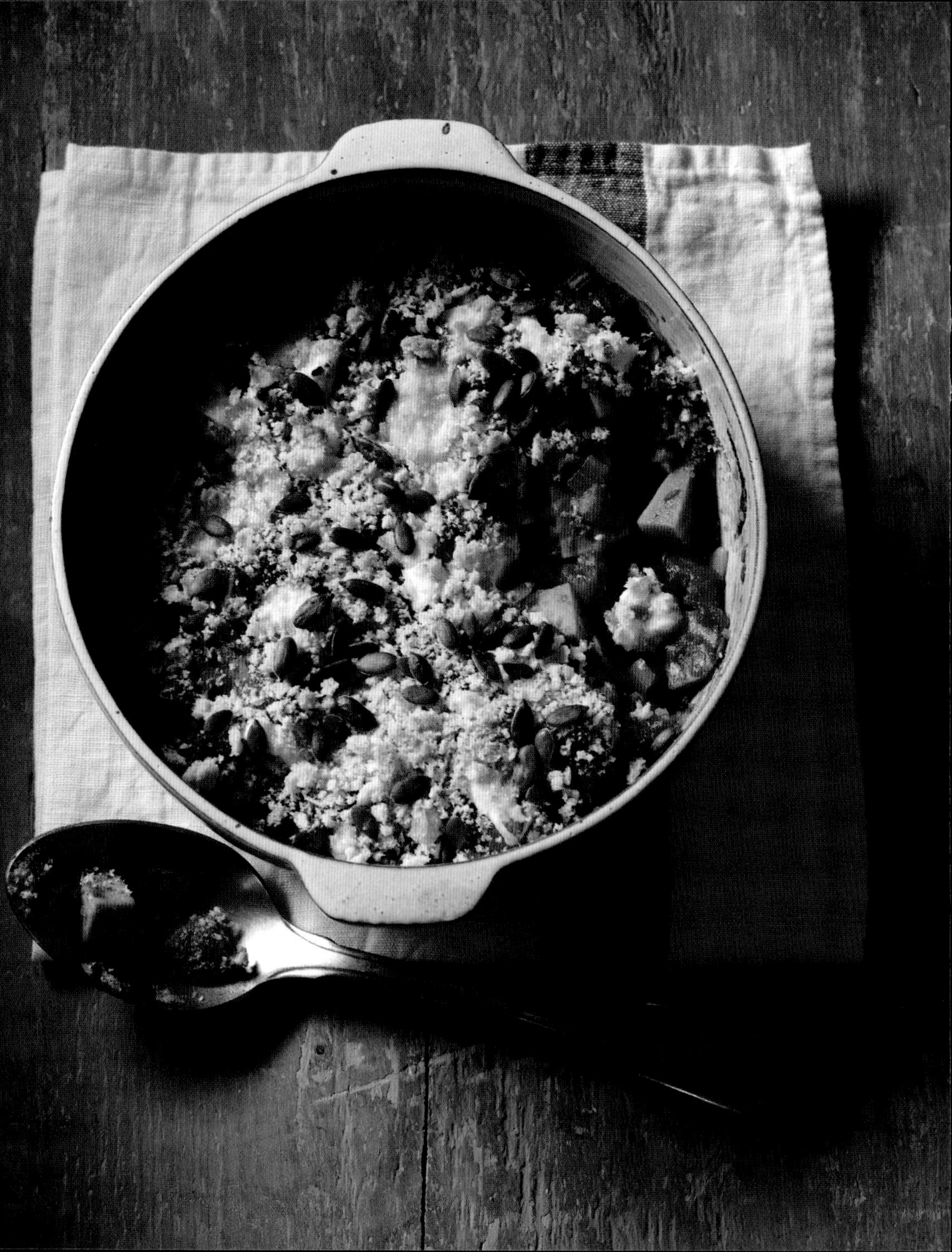

Sweet potato and pumpkin seed cheesy bake

Tomatoes contain the phytonutrient lycopene. Research has shown that people with low levels of lycopene often have problems falling asleep. This bake combines sleep-friendly sweet potatoes, pumpkin seeds and cheese.

SERVES 4
PREP: 10 minutes
COOK: 35–40 minutes

900 g/2 lb sweet potatoes, peeled and cubed
3 fresh thyme sprigs, leaves stripped
2 tsp cumin seeds
250 ml/9 fl oz vegetable stock
100 ml/3½ fl oz half-fat crème fraîche
120 g/4 oz soft goat's cheese, e.g. chèvre
4 tbsp pumpkin seeds
4 tbsp fresh breadcrumbs

FOR THE TOMATO SAUCE:
2 tbsp olive oil
1 large onion, finely chopped
2 garlic cloves, crushed
1 x 400 g/14 oz can chopped tomatoes
1 tbsp tomato paste
balsamic vinegar for drizzling
salt and freshly ground black pepper

Preheat the oven to 180°C/350°F/gas mark 4.

Put the sweet potatoes in a large baking dish and sprinkle with the thyme leaves and cumin seeds. Add a grinding of black pepper and pour the stock over the top. Bake in the preheated oven for 20–25 minutes or until just tender but not mushy.

Meanwhile, make the tomato sauce. Heat the oil in a large frying pan set over a low heat and cook the onion and garlic, stirring occasionally, for 8–10 minutes until softened but not coloured. Add the tomatoes and tomato paste and simmer gently for 10 minutes or until the sauce reduces and thickens. Add a dash of balsamic vinegar and season to taste with salt and pepper.

Spoon the tomato sauce over and around the sweet potatoes. Dot the top with small spoonfuls of crème fraîche and goat's cheese. Sprinkle with pumpkin seeds and breadcrumbs.

Turn up the oven to 200°C/400°F/gas mark 6 and cook for 15 minutes until the topping is crisp and golden.

Or you can try this ...

★ Use pumpkin or butternut squash instead of sweet potatoes.
★ Add chopped fresh basil, parsley, chives or rosemary.
★ Instead of canned tomatoes, use 500 g/1 lb 2 oz juicy fresh ones.

Crunchy sesame chicken

SERVES 4
PREP: 10 minutes
COOK: 10 minutes

2 tbsp soy sauce
1 tbsp hoisin sauce
1 tbsp clear honey
2 tbsp sesame oil
a pinch of salt
4 thick chicken breast fillets, skinned and cut into thick slices
100 g/3½ oz white or black sesame seeds
2.5 cm/1 in piece fresh root ginger, peeled and shredded
2 garlic cloves, thinly sliced
1 tsp cumin seeds
1 bunch spring onions, diagonally sliced
450 g/1 lb baby spinach leaves
juice of ½ lime
steamed brown rice to serve

Sesame seeds contain vitamin B6, calcium and magnesium, which are all conducive to quality sleep. They also help to lower blood pressure and cholesterol levels, making them an extremely healthy food to include in your diet.

In a large bowl, mix together the soy and hoisin sauces, honey and one teaspoon of sesame oil. Stir in the salt and add the chicken, turning the slices in the mixture.

Spread the sesame seeds evenly in a shallow dish and use them to coat the chicken slices.

Heat one tablespoon of sesame oil in a wok or deep frying pan set over a medium heat. Add the sesame coated chicken to the hot pan and cook for 3–4 minutes each side until the pieces are browned and slightly sticky and the chicken is cooked right through.

Meanwhile, in another wok heat the remaining oil and stir-fry the ginger, garlic and cumin seeds over a medium to high heat for 2 minutes or until they start to crackle. Add the spring onions and spinach and stir-fry briskly until the spinach wilts. Stir in the lime juice.

Serve the chicken with the stir-fried spinach and some brown rice.

Or you can try this...

★ Add a dash of soy sauce or nam pla (Thai fish sauce) to the spinach.
★ Add some fine green beans or torn pack choi (bok choy) to the stir-fry.
★ Serve with rice noodles or even some quinoa.

Steak and mushrooms with sweet potato 'fries'

Chimichurri is a tangy green uncooked sauce that's widely eaten throughout South America. The fresh herbs are a great way of boosting your daily intake of vitamins and minerals.

SERVES 4
PREP: 15 minutes
COOK: 20–25 minutes

2 large sweet potatoes, peeled and cut into thin chips
4 tbsp olive oil, plus extra for brushing
60 g/2 oz (4 tbsp) unsalted butter
450 g/1 lb mushrooms, e.g. white, chestnut or wild
4 lean sirloin or fillet steaks
salt and freshly ground black pepper

FOR THE CHIMICHURRI:
1 small bunch fresh flat-leaf parsley, finely chopped
a handful of fresh coriander, chopped
4 fresh oregano sprigs, leaves stripped
3 garlic cloves, crushed
1 shallot, finely chopped
½ tsp smoked paprika
3 tbsp fruity green olive oil
1 tbsp red wine vinegar
juice of ½ lemon
sea salt crystals and freshly ground black pepper

Preheat the oven to 190°C/375°F/gas mark 5.

In a bowl, stir the sweet potatoes in two tablespoons of olive oil, turning them until they are lightly coated all over. Season with salt and pepper.

Transfer the sweet potatoes to a large baking sheet, spreading them out. Cook in the preheated oven for about 20 minutes until the fries are crisp and golden brown.

Meanwhile, make the chimichurri: mix all the ingredients together in a bowl or blitz in a blender for a smoother sauce.

Heat the butter and remaining olive oil in a frying pan set over a medium heat. Add the mushrooms and cook for 5 minutes or so until tender and golden brown on both sides.

When the sweet potato fries are nearly ready, brush the steaks lightly with oil and season with salt and pepper. Heat a ridged griddle pan over a medium to high heat and add the steaks. Cook for 2–4 minutes on each side, depending on how well cooked you like your steak. They should be slightly charred on the outside but pink and juicy inside.

Place a steak and some mushrooms on each serving plate and spoon the chimichurri over the top. Serve immediately with the hot sweet potato fries.

Sicilian spaghetti with sardines

SERVES 4
PREP: 5 minutes
COOK: 10–12 minutes

- 500 g/1 lb 2 oz wholemeal spaghetti (dry weight)
- 2 x 120 g/4 oz cans sardines in olive oil
- 2 garlic cloves, crushed
- 2 tsp fennel seeds
- 4 tbsp pine nuts
- 2 tbsp capers, drained
- 4 tbsp sultanas
- juice of ½ lemon
- a dash of balsamic vinegar
- a handful of fresh parsley, finely chopped
- freshly ground black pepper

This *agrodolce* (sweet and sour) pasta dish, which is typical of Sicilian cooking, is quick, easy and economical to make. Like other oily fish, sardines are very healthy and rich in vitamins B6 and D, calcium, magnesium and potassium.

Cook the spaghetti according to the instructions on the packet. Drain well, reserving some of the cooking liquid.

Meanwhile, heat one tablespoon of oil from the sardines in a frying pan over a low heat. Add the garlic and fennel seeds and cook for 2 minutes without browning.

Drain the remaining sardines and add to the pan with the pine nuts, capers and sultanas. Heat through gently, stirring once or twice and breaking up the sardines a little into smaller pieces.

Add the sardine mixture to the drained spaghetti and stir in the lemon juice, a little of the reserved pasta cooking liquid, a dash of balsamic vinegar and the parsley. Season with black pepper.

Divide the spaghetti between four bowls and serve immediately.

Or you can try this…

★ Stir in some rocket or baby spinach leaves at the end just before serving so they wilt into the pasta.
★ Add some chopped onion or fennel bulb.
★ Sprinkle with toasted fresh wholemeal breadcrumbs just before serving.

Prawn and spinach linguine

Prawns contain tryptophan which is calming and sedating. When tryptophan-rich foods are eaten with healthy carbs – like the wholemeal linguine in this recipe – tryptophan is better absorbed into the bloodstream, helping the body move towards sleep.

SERVES 4
PREP: 5 minutes
COOK: 10–12 minutes

500 g/1 lb 2 oz wholemeal linguine (dry weight)
2 tbsp olive oil
4 garlic cloves, crushed
1 bunch fresh parsley, finely chopped
grated zest and juice of 1 large lemon
120 ml/4 fl oz white wine
400 g/14 oz raw peeled large prawns
300 g/10 oz baby spinach leaves
salt and freshly ground black pepper

Cook the linguine according to the instructions on the packet until just tender (*al dente*). Drain well.

Meanwhile, heat the oil in a large deep frying pan set over a low heat. Cook the garlic, without browning, for 1 minute. Add half the parsley, the lemon zest and juice and the wine, then turn up the heat and let the sauce bubble away for about 5 minutes until it reduces.

Add the prawns and cook for 1–2 minutes until they turn pink underneath, then turn them over and quickly cook the other side. Do not overcook them or they will be dry and less juicy and succulent. Stir in the remaining parsley and the spinach, then season to taste.

Add the cooked linguine to the pan and gently toss everything together. Divide between four warm serving plates and serve immediately.

Or you can try this…

★ Use any gluten-free pasta: spaghetti, tagliatelle or pasta shapes.
★ Instead of parsley, try chives, basil or coriander.
★ Rocket or shredded greens can be substituted for the spinach.

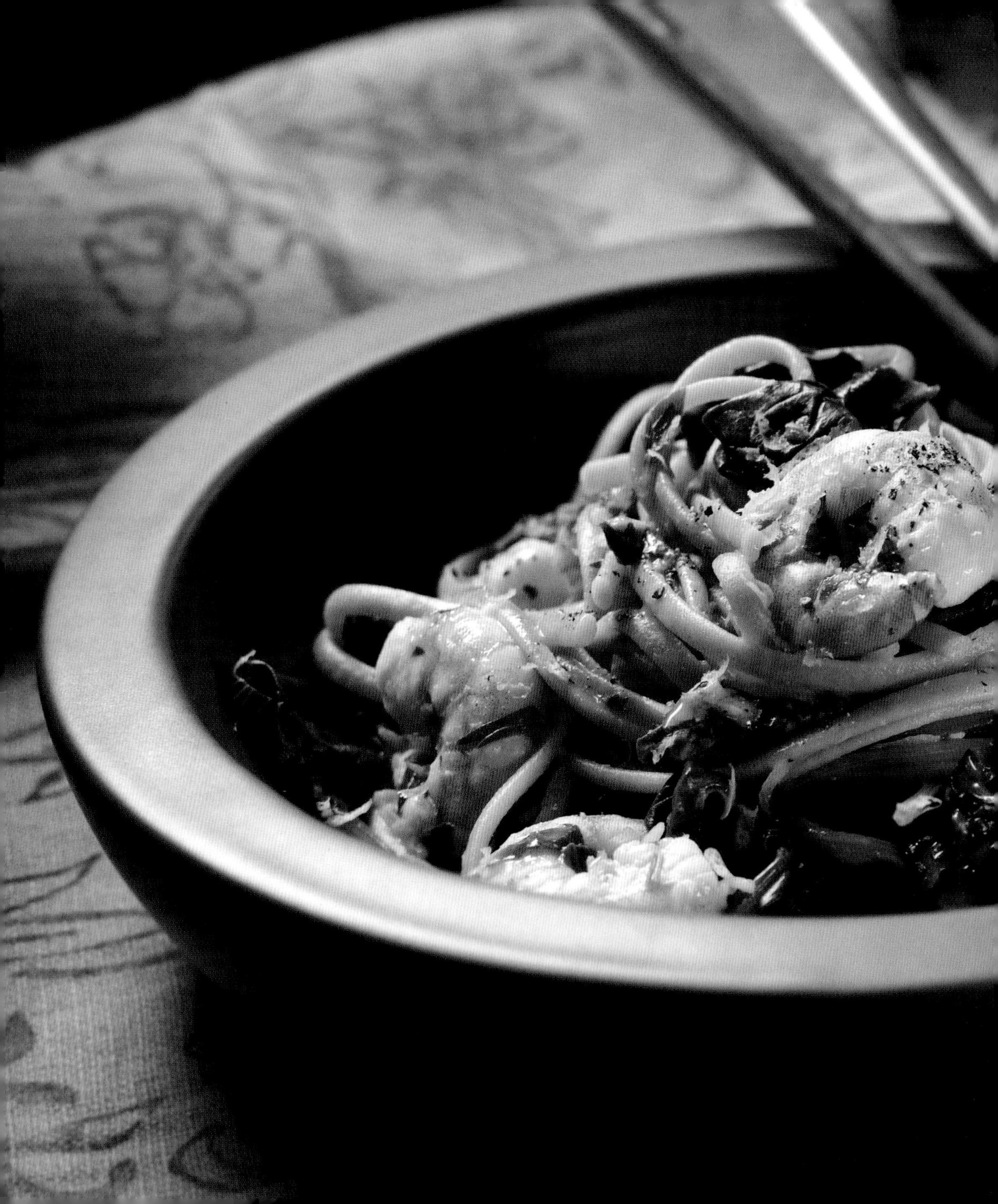

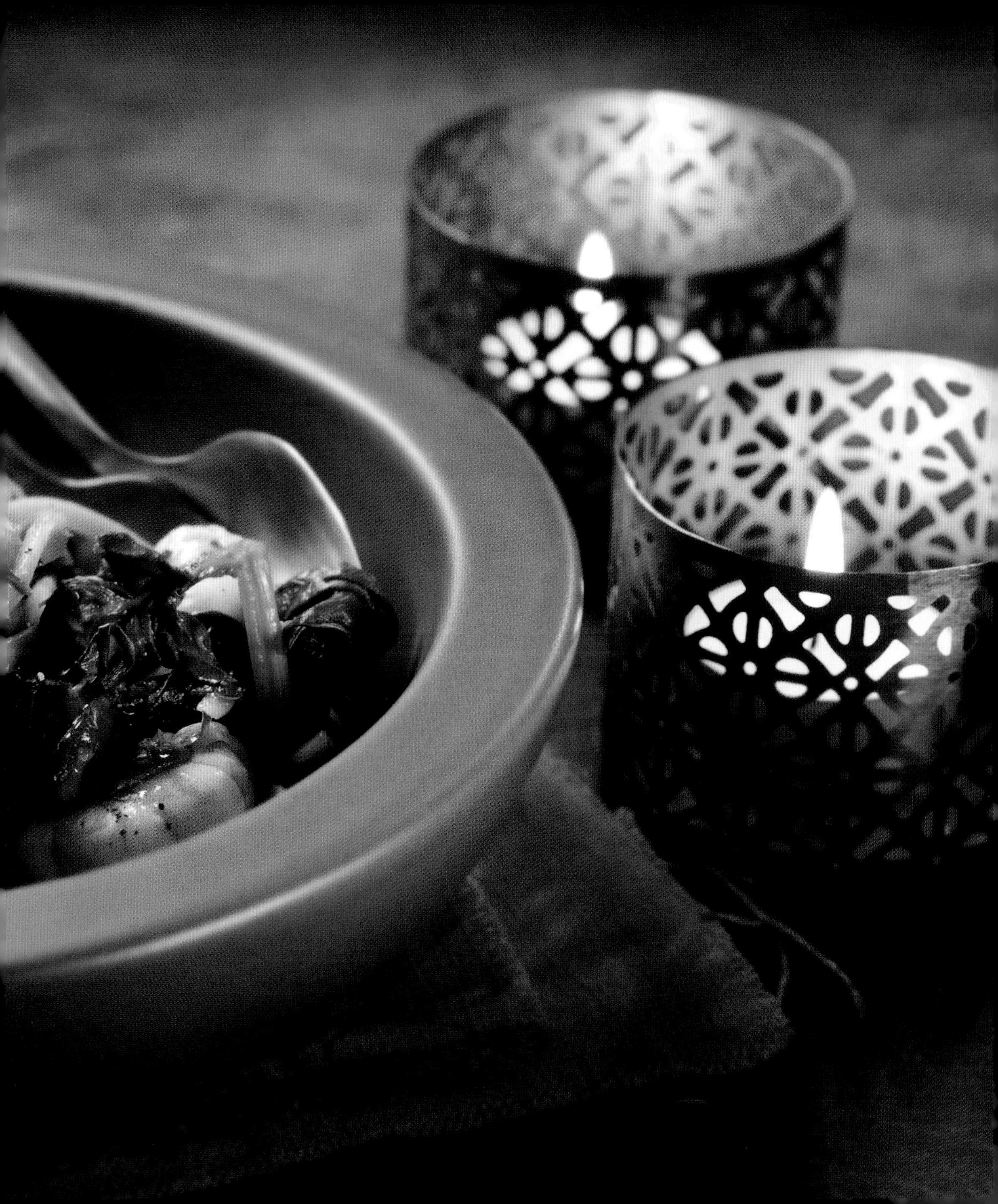

Creamy wild mushroom and spinach fettuccine

SERVES 4
PREP: 10 minutes
COOK: 15 minutes

400 g / 14 oz fettuccine (dry weight)
2 tbsp olive oil
30 g / 1 oz (2 tbsp) butter
2 leeks, cleaned, trimmed and thinly sliced
2 garlic cloves, crushed
400 g / 14 oz wild mushrooms, sliced
240 ml / 8 fl oz crème fraîche
450 g / 1 lb spinach, washed and thick stems trimmed
salt and freshly ground black pepper
grated Parmesan cheese to serve

The spinach, cheese and cream provide the calcium we need to make the body clock hormone melatonin, while the potassium in the mushrooms is good for digestion.

Cook the pasta according to the instructions on the packet.

Meanwhile, heat the olive oil and butter in a frying pan set over a medium heat and cook the leeks, garlic and mushrooms for 8–10 minutes until tender and slightly golden.

Reduce the heat to a simmer and stir in the crème fraîche. Cook gently for 2–3 minutes until creamy and hot.

Drain the pasta and stir in the spinach – it will wilt slightly and go bright green. Pour in the mushroom mixture and toss everything together. Season with salt and pepper.

Divide the pasta between four shallow serving bowls or plates and serve immediately, sprinkled with Parmesan.

Or you can try this...

★ If you can't get wild mushrooms, use chestnut, white mushrooms or even oriental ones.
★ Substitute rocket for the spinach.

Japanese griddled tuna with rice

Like salmon, tuna is a great source of the sleep-friendly vitamins B6 and D. You should try to eat at least two helpings of oily fish every week as it also contains omega-3 fatty acids which help to keep your heart healthy.

SERVES 4
PREP: 15 minutes
COOK: 15–20 minutes

225 g/8 oz brown rice (dry weight)
120 g/4 oz frozen edamame beans
1 bunch spring onions, sliced diagonally
sunflower oil for brushing or spraying
4 fresh tuna steaks
1 sheet ready-toasted sushi nori, cut into thin shreds
2 tbsp toasted black or white sesame seeds

FOR THE JAPANESE DRESSING:
2 tbsp sunflower oil
2 tbsp toasted sesame oil
1 tbsp miso paste
1 tbsp rice vinegar
1 tbsp soy sauce
juice of ½ lime
1 garlic clove, crushed
2 tsp grated fresh root ginger
1 tsp clear honey

Cook the brown rice according to the instructions on the packet.

Meanwhile, add the beans to a pan of boiling water and cook for 3 minutes. Drain and refresh under running cold water. Drain and set aside.

Whisk together all the ingredients for the Japanese dressing.

Gently stir the rice with a fork to separate the grains. Mix in the cooked beans and the spring onions. Add the Japanese dressing and toss them all gently together.

Lightly brush or spray a non-stick griddle pan with oil and place over a medium to high heat. Add the tuna and cook for 2–3 minutes on each side, depending on how well cooked you like it.

Divide the rice mixture between four serving plates and top with the tuna steaks. Sprinkle with the shredded nori and sesame seeds and serve.

Or you can try this …

★ Top the rice with griddled chicken or tofu.
★ Use canned beans of your choice instead of edamame.
★ Brush the tuna with some of the Japanese dressing before griddling it.

Stir-fried quinoa and cashews

SERVES 4
PREP: 15 minutes
COOK: 20 minutes

60 g/2 oz cashews
480 ml/16 fl oz vegetable stock
200 g/7 oz quinoa (dry weight)
250 g/9 oz broccoli, cut into florets
150 g/5 oz mangetout, trimmed
2 tbsp olive oil
1 bunch spring onions, sliced
1 red pepper, deseeded and diced
2 garlic cloves, crushed
2.5 cm/1 in piece fresh root ginger, peeled and diced
½ tsp ground coriander
3 tbsp light soy sauce
grated zest and juice of 1 lemon
200 g/7 oz baby plum tomatoes, quartered
salt and freshly ground black pepper
a handful of fresh coriander, chopped

Quinoa is a good source of calcium and tryptophan and cashews contain sleep-enhancing calcium, magnesium, potassium, vitamin B6 and tryptophan.

Set a small frying pan over a medium heat. Add the cashews and gently toss them for 1–2 minutes until golden brown. Remove from the pan immediately before they catch and burn and set aside.

Heat the stock in a saucepan and when it starts to boil add the quinoa. Cover and simmer gently for 15 minutes until tender, most of the liquid has been absorbed and the 'sprout' pops out of each seed. Remove from the heat and leave to steam in the pan for 5 minutes before draining and fluffing up with a fork.

Meanwhile, blanch the broccoli in a pan of boiling water for 1 minute. Plunge into a bowl of iced water to cool, then drain. Repeat with the mangetout.

Heat the oil in a wok or deep frying pan over a medium heat and stir-fry the spring onions, red pepper, garlic and ginger for 2 minutes. Stir in the ground coriander, soy sauce, lemon zest and juice, tomatoes, broccoli and mangetout. Stir-fry briskly for 2 minutes, then add the quinoa and cook for 1 minute. Season to taste with salt and pepper.

Divide between four bowls and serve sprinkled with the cashews and coriander.

Or you can try this...

- Instead of cashews, try walnuts, almonds, pistachios or hazelnuts.
- Add some seeds: pumpkin, cumin or fennel.
- For the stir-fried vegetables try courgettes, fennel, mushrooms or green or yellow peppers.

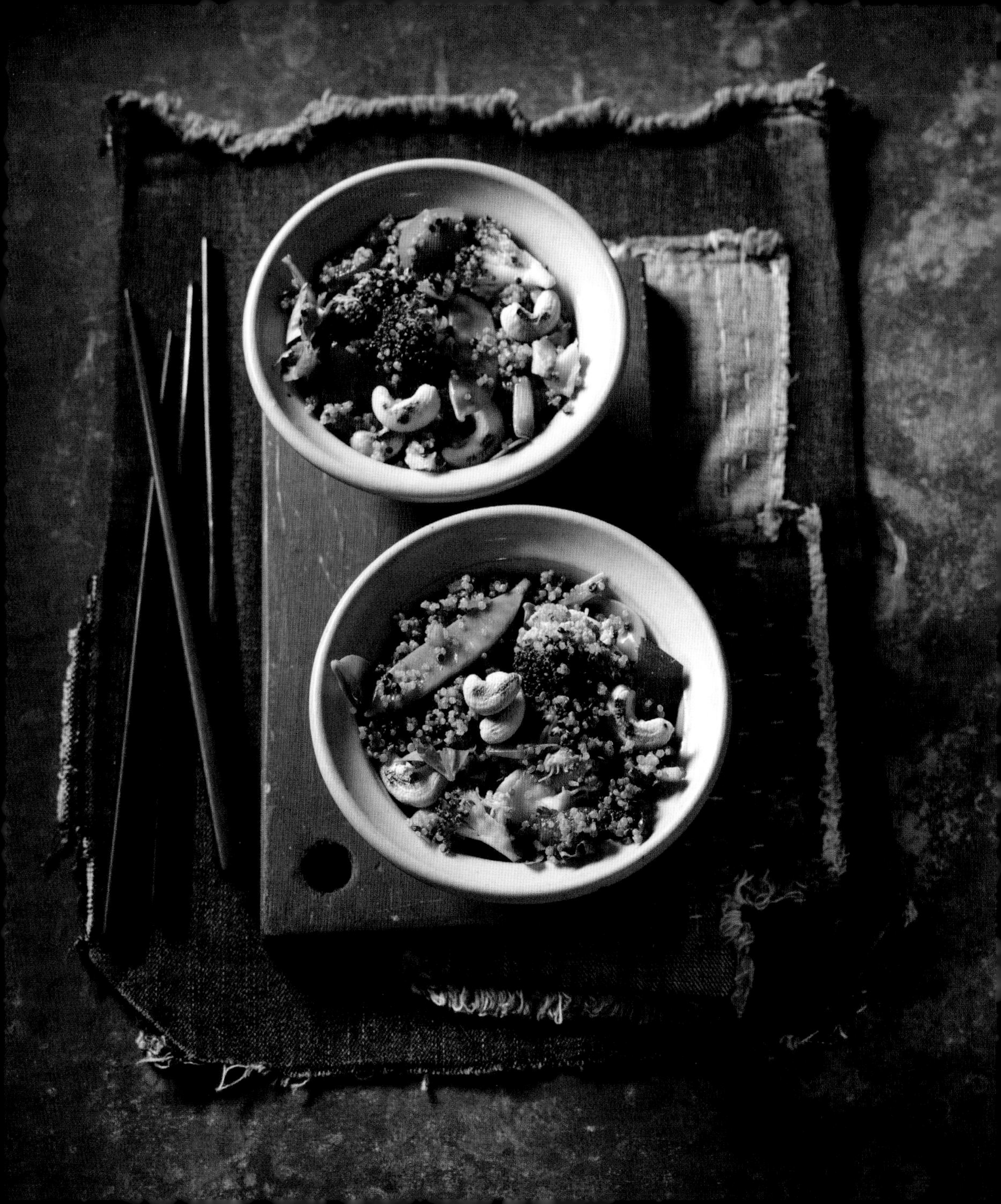

Spaghetti carbonara with mushrooms

SERVES 4
PREP: 10 minutes
COOK: 10–15 minutes

1 tbsp olive oil
2 garlic cloves, thinly sliced
150 g/5 oz pancetta or bacon, cubed
300 g/10 oz mushrooms, sliced
30 g/1 oz butter
500 g/1 lb 2 oz spaghetti (dry weight)
2 large eggs and 2 yolks
60 ml/2 fl oz crème fraîche or double cream
85 g/3 oz grated Parmesan cheese, plus extra to serve
salt and freshly ground black pepper

This Roman speciality is such a soothing supper and so easy to cook with minimal preparation. The mushrooms contain vitamin D, which targets the part of our brain associated with sleep, while the dairy foods are rich in tryptophan.

Heat the oil in a large saucepan set over a low to medium heat and cook the garlic for a couple of minutes until it colours. Remove immediately and discard. Add the pancetta or bacon to the pan and cook for about 5 minutes, turning occasionally, until golden and most of the fat has run out. Remove from the heat.

Cook the mushrooms in the butter in a frying pan set over a medium heat, turning and stirring, until golden brown. Add to the pan containing the pancetta.

Meanwhile, cook the spaghetti according to the instructions on the packet until it's tender but still slightly firm (*al dente*).

Beat the eggs, yolks, crème fraîche and grated cheese together in a bowl. Add a grinding of black pepper.

Drain the pasta, reserving a ladleful of the cooking water. Add the pasta to the pan containing the pancetta and stir well. Stir in the egg and cheese mixture. Keep stirring and tossing the pasta off the heat until the egg mixtures thickens and is creamy. If it's too thick and needs some moisture, add a little of the reserved pasta cooking liquid. Check the seasoning, adding salt if required.

Divide the pasta between four warm shallow serving bowls. Sprinkle with more Parmesan if wished.

Creamy mushroom and butterbean gratin

Mushrooms, beans and dairy products (milk and cheese) are all good to eat before going to bed as they can relieve insomnia and promote healthy sleep.

SERVES 4
PREP: 15 minutes
COOK: 45–55 minutes

3 tbsp olive oil, plus extra for drizzling
1 large onion, chopped
2 garlic cloves, crushed
500 g/1 lb 2 oz mushrooms, quartered or sliced
2 x 4 00g/14 oz can butterbeans, rinsed and drained
1 small bunch fresh parsley, finely chopped
60 g/2 oz fresh wholemeal breadcrumbs
60 g/2 oz grated Parmesan cheese

FOR THE WHITE SAUCE:
60 g/2 oz butter
60 g/2 oz plain flour
480 ml/16 fl oz milk
a pinch of ground nutmeg
salt and freshly ground black pepper

Preheat the oven to 180°C/350°F/gas mark 4.

Heat the oil in a saucepan set over a low heat. Add the onion and garlic and cook for 6–8 minutes, stirring occasionally, until tender but not coloured.

Add the mushrooms and cook, stirring occasionally, for about 5 minutes until tender and golden.

Meanwhile, make the white sauce: melt the butter in a non-stick pan set over a low heat and stir in the flour with a wooden spoon. Cook for 2 minutes until it smells 'biscuity' and then add the milk, a little at a time, stirring or whisking until smooth. Keep stirring over a low heat until the sauce thickens. Remove from the heat and season with the nutmeg, salt and pepper.

Add the butterbeans, parsley and white sauce to the onion and mushroom mixture and stir gently. Transfer to a baking dish.

Sprinkle the breadcrumbs and cheese over the top and drizzle with a little oil. Bake in the preheated oven for 30–40 minutes until crisp and golden brown and bubbling around the edges.

Serve hot with some steamed or boiled green vegetables.

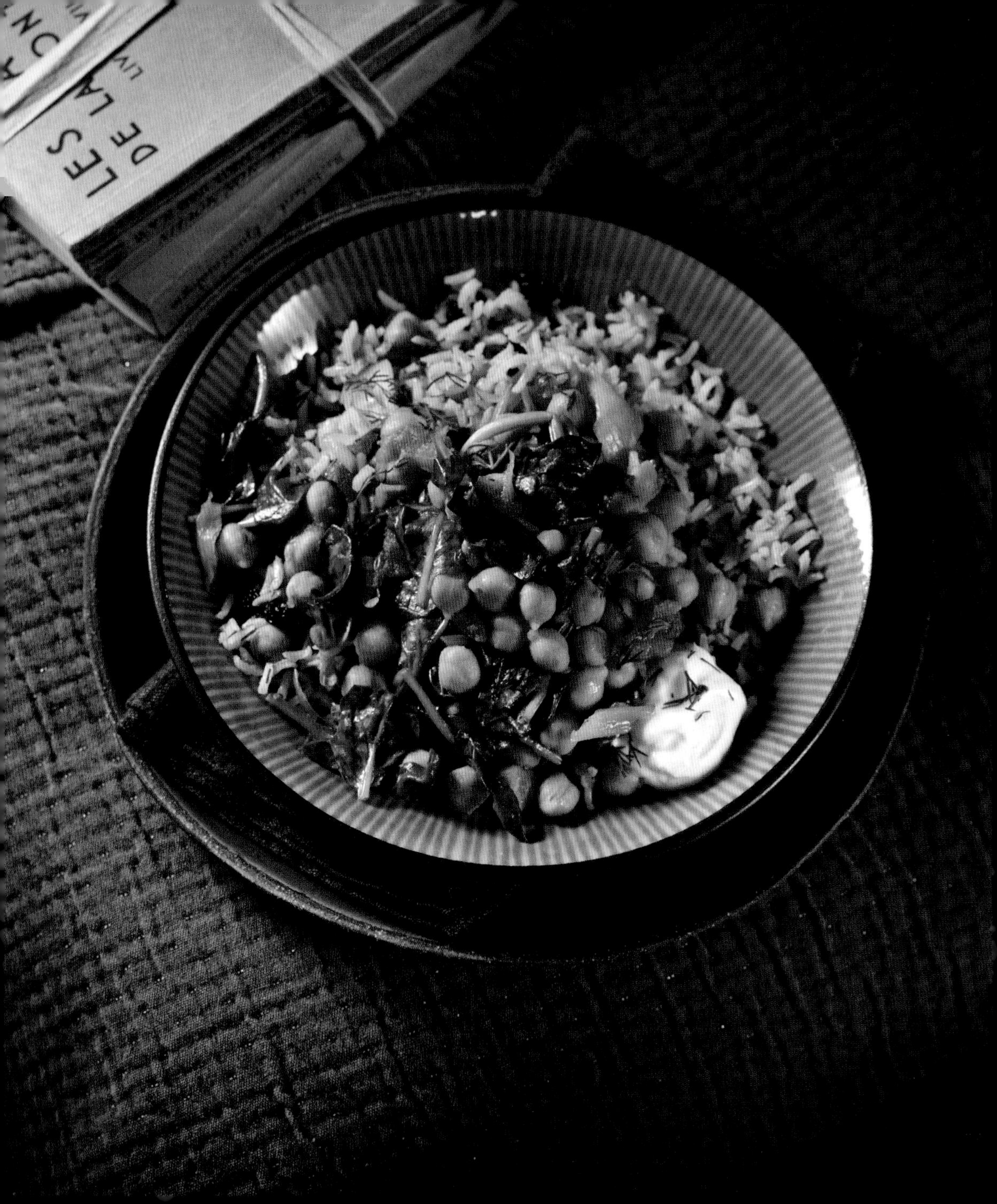
LES

Greek rice pilaf with lemony greens, dill and chickpeas

You can serve this warm as a veggie supper or with grilled fish, lamb or chicken. The brown rice and chickpeas are both good sources of tryptophan and have a natural sedative effect.

SERVES 4
PREP: 15 minutes
COOK: 30 minutes

90 ml/3 fl oz olive oil
1 bunch spring onions, finely sliced
2 garlic cloves, crushed
1 tsp ground cumin
½ tsp ground coriander
1 tsp paprika
4 tomatoes, skinned and chopped
2 x 400 g/14 oz cans chickpeas, rinsed and drained
1 kg/1 lb 2 oz spinach, washed, trimmed and chopped
1 small bunch fresh dill, finely chopped
juice of 1 large lemon
salt and freshly ground black pepper
Greek yoghurt to serve

FOR THE RICE PILAF:
2 tbsp olive oil
1 small onion, finely chopped
225 g/8 oz brown rice (dry weight)
1 tsp paprika
480 ml/16 fl oz chicken stock
juice of 1 lemon
1 long strip of lemon zest
a handful of fresh dill, chopped
4 tbsp currants

Make the rice pilaf: heat the olive oil in a heavy-based pan over a low to medium heat and cook the onion, stirring occasionally, for 6–8 minutes until tender. Add the rice and cook for 1–2 minutes, stirring all the time. Stir in the paprika and then add the chicken stock, lemon juice and zest and bring to the boil. Reduce the heat, cover with a lid and simmer gently for 20 minutes until the rice is cooked and has absorbed all the stock. Remove the lemon zest and add the dill and currants. Fluff up the rice with a fork.

Meanwhile, heat the olive oil in a large heavy-based saucepan and cook the spring onions and garlic over a low heat, stirring occasionally, for about 5 minutes, until tender.

Stir in the ground spices and paprika and cook for 1 minute. Add the tomatoes and cook gently for 5 minutes. Stir in the chickpeas and spinach and cook gently for 3–4 minutes until the spinach wilts and the chickpeas are warmed through. Season to taste with salt and pepper, then stir in the chopped dill and lemon juice.

Divide the rice pilaf between four bowls and top with the chickpea and spinach mixture. Serve with some Greek yoghurt.

Chicken, mushrooms, greens and cashew stir-fry

SERVES 4
PREP: 10 minutes
COOK: 15 minutes

250 g/9 oz brown rice (dry weight)
2 tbsp groundnut oil
500 g/1 lb 2 oz skinned chicken breast fillets, cubed
450 g/1 lb chestnut mushrooms, quartered
2.5 cm/1 in piece fresh root ginger, peeled and diced
2 garlic cloves, crushed
4 spring onions , sliced
200 g/7 oz kale, ribs and stalks removed, leaves shredded
2 tbsp soy sauce
2–3 tbsp hot chicken stock
120 g/4 oz roasted cashews

This really speedy supper is delicious. The mushrooms are a good way to top up your vitamin D levels – the vitamin that targets the neurons in the brain associated with sleep. Researchers think that people who have a vitamin D deficiency may have sleep disorders.

Cook the rice according to the packet instructions.

Meanwhile, heat the oil in a wok or large deep frying pan set over a medium to high heat. Add the chicken and stir-fry briskly for 5 minutes until slightly browned all over.

Add the mushrooms, ginger, garlic and spring onions and stir-fry for 2 minutes.

Add the kale and stir-fry for 2–3 minutes. Moisten with the soy sauce and chicken stock and stir in the cashews.

Serve immediately with the boiled rice.

Or you can try this ...

★ Use shredded spring greens or Savoy cabbage instead of kale.
★ Add thinly sliced red and yellow peppers or carrot matchsticks.
★ Serve with boiled eggs or rice noodles or even some quinoa.
★ Any mushrooms can be used.

Oat-crusted fishcakes

You can make these fishcakes in advance and freeze them until required. Mackerel and oats are a winning combination flavourwise, nutritionally and for encouraging quality sleep.

SERVES 4
PREP: 20 minutes
CHILL: 20–30 minutes
COOK: 25 minutes

675 g/1½ lb potatoes, peeled and cut into chunks
15 g/½ oz butter
300 g/10 oz smoked mackerel, skinned and flaked
1 bunch spring onions, finely chopped
1 small bunch fresh parsley, finely chopped
grated zest and juice of 1 small lemon
1 large free-range egg, beaten
120 g/4 oz rolled oats or pinhead oatmeal
olive oil for shallow frying
salt and freshly ground black pepper
lemon wedges to serve

FOR THE HORSERADISH SAUCE:
180 ml/6 fl oz crème fraîche
1–2 tbsp creamed horseradish
a handful of fresh dill, chopped
a squeeze of lemon juice

Cook the potatoes in a large pan of boiling water until tender but not mushy. Drain well and mash with the butter until smooth.

Add the smoked mackerel, spring onions, parsley, lemon zest and juice. Season lightly with salt and pepper. Divide into eight portions and shape each one into a patty with your hands.

Dip the fishcakes into the beaten egg and then coat them lightly with the oats. Cover and chill in the fridge for 20–30 minutes to firm them up.

Heat the olive oil in a large frying pan set over a medium heat and cook the fishcakes, in batches, for 4–5 minutes each side until crisp and golden brown.

Meanwhile, mix together all the ingredients for the creamy horseradish sauce in a bowl.

Serve the fishcakes and creamy horseradish sauce with lemon wedges and some salad or green vegetables.

Or you can try this …

★ Use drained canned sardines in oil instead of mackerel, or smoked salmon.
★ Add some mayonnaise to the horseradish sauce.
★ Add some chopped dill and capers to the fishcake mixture.

Seared teriyaki salmon with stir-fried broccoli noodles

SERVES 4
PREP: 10 minutes
COOK: 10–15 minutes

4 salmon fillets
250 g/9 oz egg noodles (dry weight)
2 tbsp toasted sesame oil
1 bunch spring onions sliced
300 g/10 oz broccoli, cut into small florets
300 g/10 oz mushrooms, quartered or sliced
1 tbsp sesame seeds

FOR THE TERIYAKI SAUCE:
4 tbsp soy sauce
4 tsp mirin
1 tbsp clear honey
1 tbsp diced fresh root ginger
2 garlic cloves, crushed

A really easy supper for when you arrive home tired after a busy day at work and don't want to spend a long time in the kitchen. The salmon, sesame seeds and soy are all good sources of tryptophan.

Make the teriyaki sauce: mix all the ingredients together and brush a little over the salmon fillets.

Cook the egg noodles according to the instructions on the packet. Drain well.

While the noodles are cooking, heat one tablespoon of the toasted sesame oil in a frying pan over a medium heat. Add the salmon fillets to the hot pan and cook for about 3 minutes on each side until golden brown and cooked right through.

Meanwhile, heat the remaining toasted sesame oil in a wok or deep frying pan set over a high heat. Add the spring onions, broccoli and mushrooms and stir-fry for 4–5 minutes until they are just tender but still retain some bite.

Stir in the remaining teriyaki sauce and the cooked noodles. Heat through for 2 minutes and then divide the mixture between four plates.

Top with the salmon fillets, sprinkle with sesame seeds and serve immediately.

Or you can try this...

★ Instead of egg noodles use udon or rice noodles.
★ Omit the noodles and serve on a bed of brown rice.
★ Try making this with chicken breasts or large prawns.

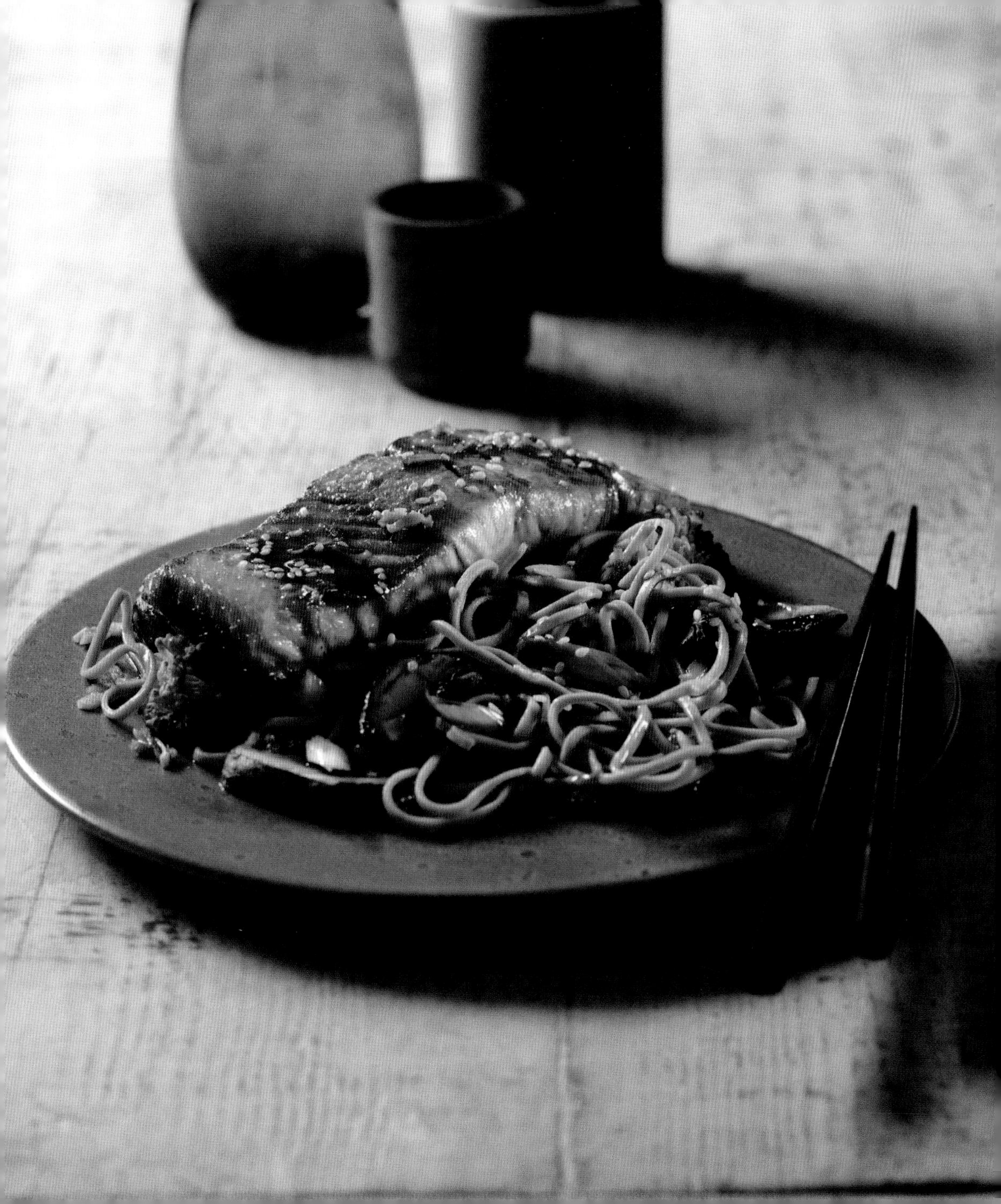

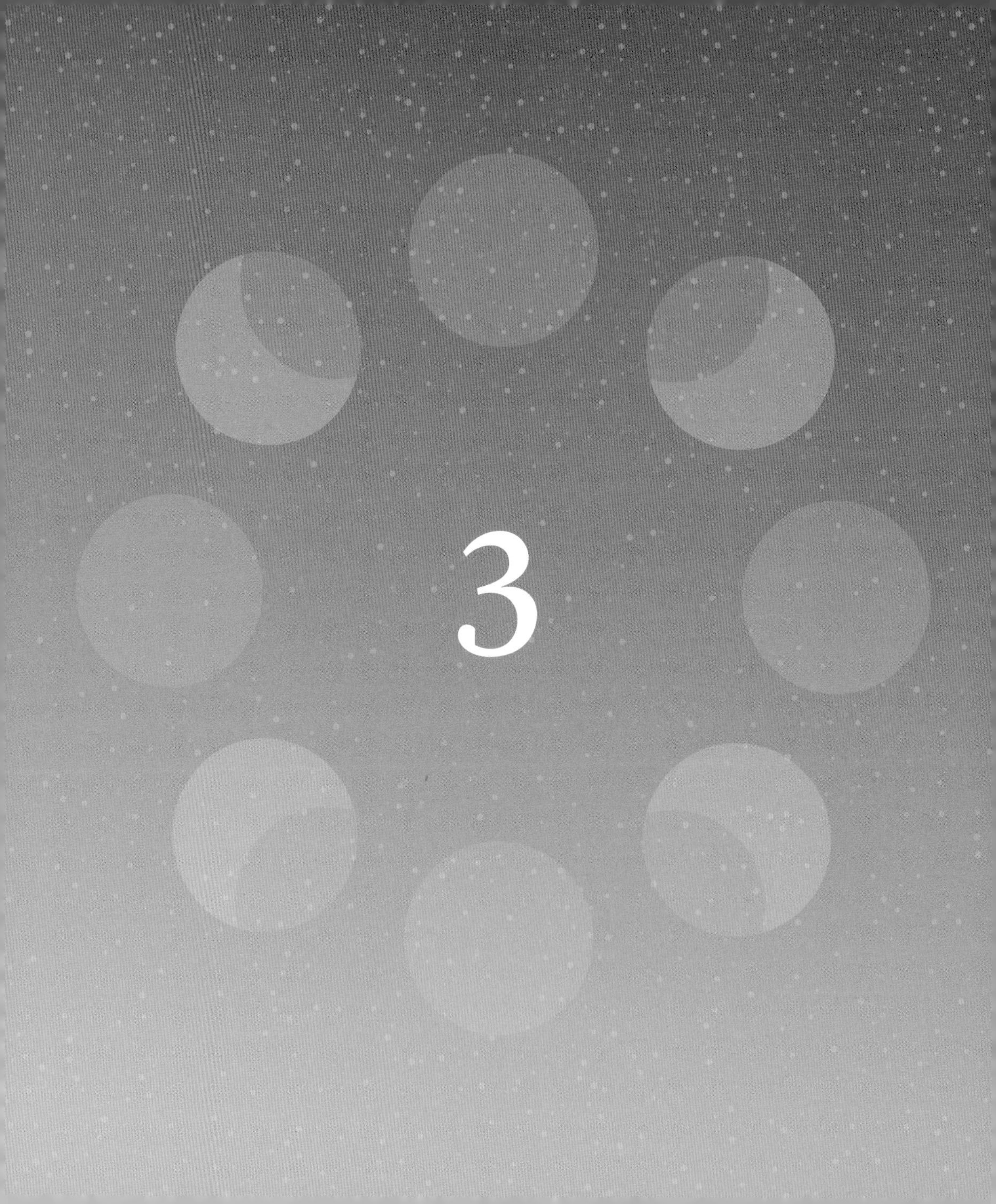

3

BAKING AND DESSERTS

Seedy fruit and nut bars

MAKES 12 BARS
PREP: 15 minutes
COOK: 35–40 minutes

- 300 g/10 oz rolled oats
- 85 g/3 oz chopped walnuts
- 100 g/3½ oz ready-to-eat dried apricots, chopped
- 100g/3½oz dried figs, chopped
- 100 g/3½ oz raisins or dried cherries
- 1 tbsp pumpkin seeds
- 1 tbsp sunflower seeds
- 1 tbsp sesame seeds
- 1 tbsp chia seeds
- 150 g/5 oz butter, plus extra for greasing
- 6 tbsp clear honey

These delicious bars are packed with nutrients and perfect for a bedtime snack. Walnuts contain their own melatonin – the hormone that sets your body clock.

Preheat the oven to 160°C/325°F/gas mark 3. Lightly butter a shallow 30 x 20 cm (12 x 8 in) baking tin and line with baking parchment.

Put the oats, walnuts, dried fruits and seeds in a large mixing bowl.

Put the butter and honey in a small pan set over a low heat, stirring until the butter melts and blends with the honey. Pour over the oat mixture and stir well until everything is thoroughly mixed. If it's too dry, add more melted butter; if it is too sticky, add more oats.

Spoon the mixture into the prepared tin and smooth the top. Bake in the preheated oven for 30–35 minutes until crisp and golden brown.

Remove and cool slightly before cutting into bars. Leave to get cold before removing from the tin and storing in an airtight container. The bars will stay fresh for four to five days.

Or you can try this ...

- ★ Instead of walnuts use hazelnuts or cashews.
- ★ Add prunes, dates, dried blueberries or sultanas.
- ★ Use linseeds, hemp or poppy seeds.
- ★ Stir in some crunchy peanut butter.

Chocolate, cherry, oat and almond bars

These crunchy snack bars are a real treat – and surprisingly healthy too. Cherries boost melatonin levels and relieve insomnia, while the bananas provide magnesium, potassium, vitamin B6 and tryptophan.

MAKES 8 BARS
PREP: 15 minutes
COOK: 25 minutes
CHILL: 1 hour

45 g/1½ oz ground almonds
60 g/2 oz rolled oats
a pinch of salt
150 g/5 oz almonds, coarsely chopped
60 g/2 oz dried cherries
60 g/2 oz plain chocolate, chopped
1 tbsp chia seeds
90 ml/3 fl oz clear honey
1 tbsp almond butter

Preheat the oven to 160°C/325°F/gas mark 3. Line a buttered 20 x 20 cm (8 x 8 in) baking tin with baking parchment.

Put the ground almonds, oats, salt, chopped almonds, cherries, chocolate and chia seeds in a bowl and mix together well.

Heat the honey and almond better gently in a pan set over a very low heat, stirring until blended and warm. Pour over the dry ingredients and mix thoroughly until everything is moist and coated with the honey.

Spoon into the prepared tin and level the top, pressing down well.

Bake in the preheated oven for 20 minutes until golden brown. Remove and leave to cool. When it's completely cold, cut into eight bars, and then chill in the fridge for 1 hour until set hard. Keep them in a sealed container in the fridge for up to five days.

Or you can try this...

★ Add cacao nibs and sesame seeds or ground flaxseeds.
★ Try using dried cranberries, blueberries or raisins.
★ Flavour with a few drops of vanilla extract.

Multi-seed loaf

MAKES 1 X 500 G/1 LB 2OZ LOAF
PREP: 15 minutes
STAND: 20–30 minutes
COOK: 1–1¼ hours

250 g/9 oz wholemeal flour
100 g/3½ oz porridge oats
60 g/2 oz ground flaxseed
a pinch of salt
30 g/1 oz pumpkin seeds
30 g/1 oz sunflower seeds
60 g/2 oz linseeds
2 tbsp sesame seeds
1 tsp ground cinnamon
a good pinch of grated nutmeg
100 g/3½ oz raisins
100 g/3½ oz chopped dates
60 g/2 oz chopped walnuts, plus extra for sprinkling
300 ml/½ pint skimmed milk or almond milk
2 medium free-range eggs
1 tbsp malt extract

This high-fibre loaf is quick to make as it doesn't use yeast. It's great to eat for a pre-bedtime snack as it contains calcium, potassium, magnesium, vitamins B6 and D and the essential amino acid tryptophan – a sextet of sleep-friendly nutrients.

Preheat the oven to 190°C/375°F/gas mark 5. Lightly oil a 500 g/1 lb 2oz loaf tin and line with baking parchment.

In a large mixing bowl, mix together the flour, oats, flaxseed and salt. Stir in the seeds, spices, raisins, dates and walnuts.

In another bowl, beat together the milk, eggs and malt extract. Stir into the dry ingredients until thoroughly combined. If the mixture is too stiff, add a little extra milk to loosen it.

Set aside to stand for 20–30 minutes, then transfer to the prepared loaf tin. Bake in the preheated oven for 1–1¼ hours or until the loaf is cooked right through. You know it's ready when a skewer inserted in the middle comes out clean.

Cool on a wire rack and serve cut into slices. This loaf will keep well for three to four days if wrapped in kitchen foil.

Or you can try this...

★ Add some caraway, fennel or cumin seeds.
★ Add some ground or freshly grated ginger, or a pinch of allspice.
★ Try chopped pecans, pistachios, almonds or hazelnuts.

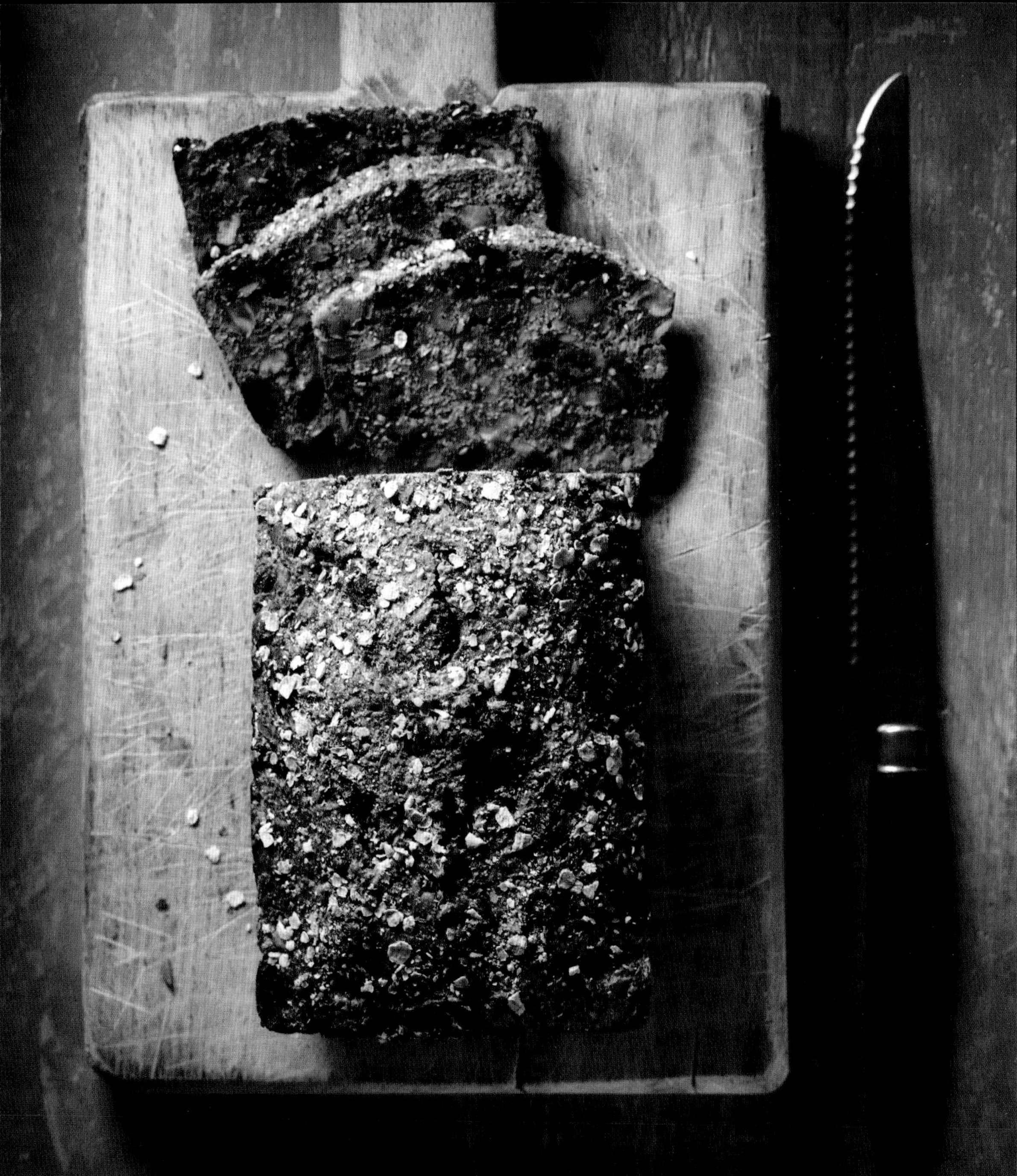

Nutty banana bread

MAKES 1 X 450 G/1 LB LOAF
PREP: 15 minutes
COOK: 1 hour

120 g/4 oz butter
175 g/6 oz light brown sugar
2 medium free-range eggs
3 large ripe bananas, mashed
150 g/5 oz coarsely chopped walnuts
225 g/8 oz self-raising flour
½ tsp bicarbonate of soda
½ tsp salt
½ tsp grated nutmeg
½ tsp ground cinnamon

This moist banana bread is deliciously satisfying and the walnuts contain melatonin to help you sleep. Bananas are a great source of vitamin B6 and tryptophan.

Preheat the oven to 180°C/350°F/gas mark 4. Line a buttered 450 g/1 lb loaf tin with baking parchment.

Cream the butter and sugar in a large bowl. Beat in the eggs, one at a time, and then mix in the mashed banana and walnuts.

Sift in the flour and bicarbonate of soda and add the salt and spices. Fold in gently.

Spoon the mixture into the prepared loaf tin and level the top. Bake in the preheated oven for about 1 hour until risen and golden brown. You can test if it's cooked by inserting a thin skewer into the centre. The banana bread is ready when the skewer comes out clean.

Leave the loaf to cool in the tin for 10 minutes and then turn out onto a wire rack. When it's cold, cut into slices to serve. It will keep well, wrapped in kitchen foil, for up to five days.

Or you can try this …

★ Add a few drops of vanilla extract.
★ Add some ground cloves, ginger or allspice.
★ Stir in some raisins or sultanas.

Cherry, oat and almond crumble

Eating cherries regularly can boost your melatonin levels, regulate your sleep cycle and help relieve insomnia. In this fabulous crumble they are combined with oats, almonds and pumpkin seeds.

SERVES 4
PREP: 15 minutes
COOK: 40–45 minutes

900 g/2 lb cherries, stoned
4 tbsp caster sugar
3 tbsp water
2 tsp cornflour
a dash of lemon juice
3 tbsp flaked almonds
crème fraîche or ice cream to serve

FOR THE CRUMBLE:
85 g/3 oz butter
150 g/5 oz plain flour
60 g/2 oz rolled oats
4 tbsp ground almonds
60 g/2 oz brown sugar
2 tbsp pumpkin seeds

Preheat the oven to 180°C/350°F/gas mark 4.

Put the cherries, sugar and water in a saucepan over a low heat and stir until the sugar dissolves. Bring to the boil, reduce the heat and simmer gently for 10 minutes until the cherries are tender and release some of their juice.

In a small bowl, stir the cornflour into a little of the cherry juices until smooth and free of lumps. Add to the cherries in the pan and stir with a wooden spoon until it starts to thicken. Add lemon juice to taste and spoon into a baking dish.

To make the crumble, cut the butter into small pieces and rub into the flour with your fingertips until it resembles fine breadcrumbs. Stir in the oats, ground almonds, sugar and pumpkin seeds. Sprinkle with two to three teaspoons of cold water and give it a stir to create some small clumps.

Spoon the crumble over the cherries right up to the edge of the dish. Sprinkle with the flaked almonds.

Bake in the preheated oven for 30–35 minutes until the crumble is crisp and golden brown and the fruit is bubbling around the edges. Serve hot with crème fraîche or ice cream.

Or you can try this…

★ Add some chopped walnuts or hazelnuts to the crumble mixture.
★ Add some ground ginger or cinnamon to the crumble mixture.
★ When cherries are out of season use apples or pears.

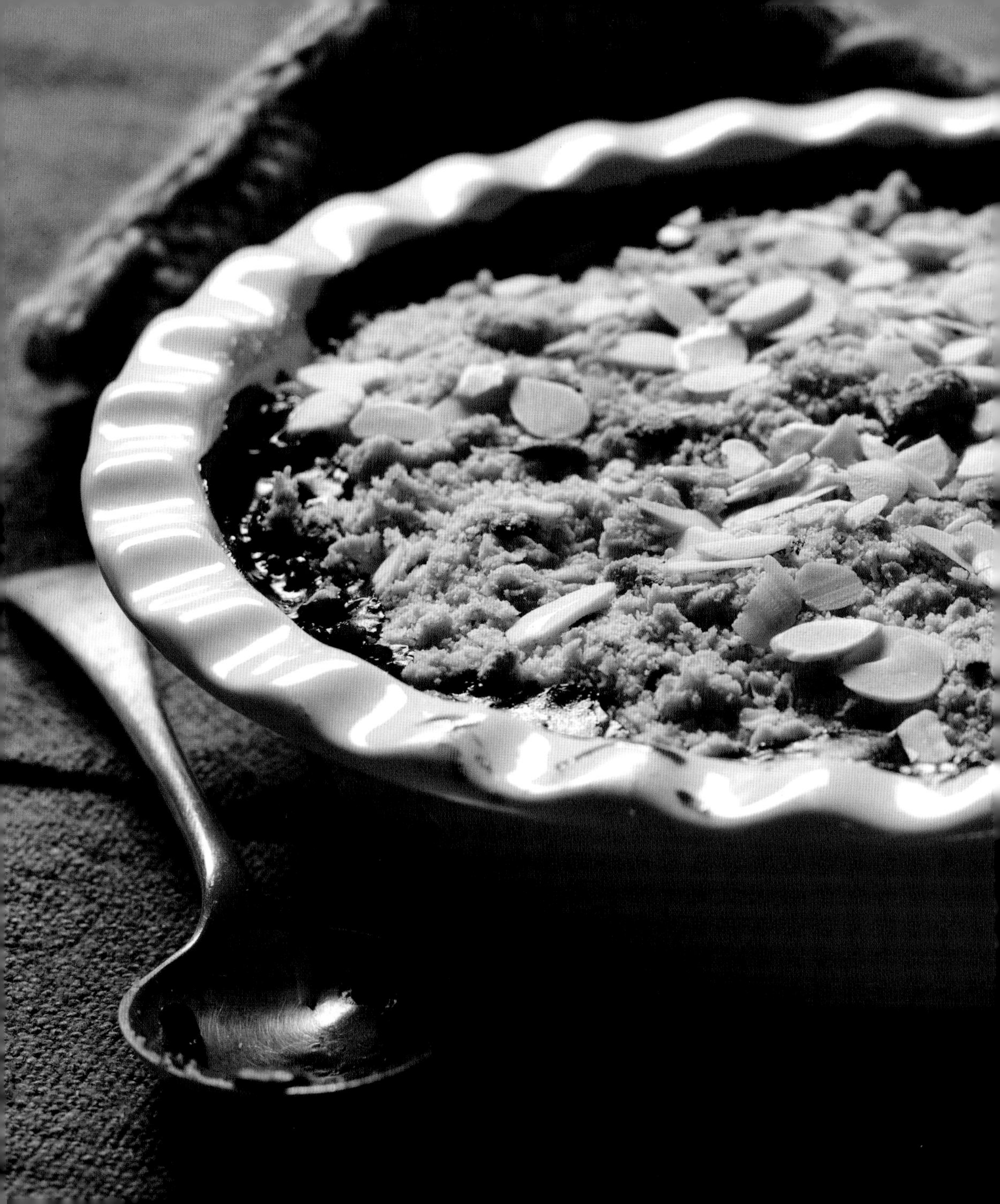

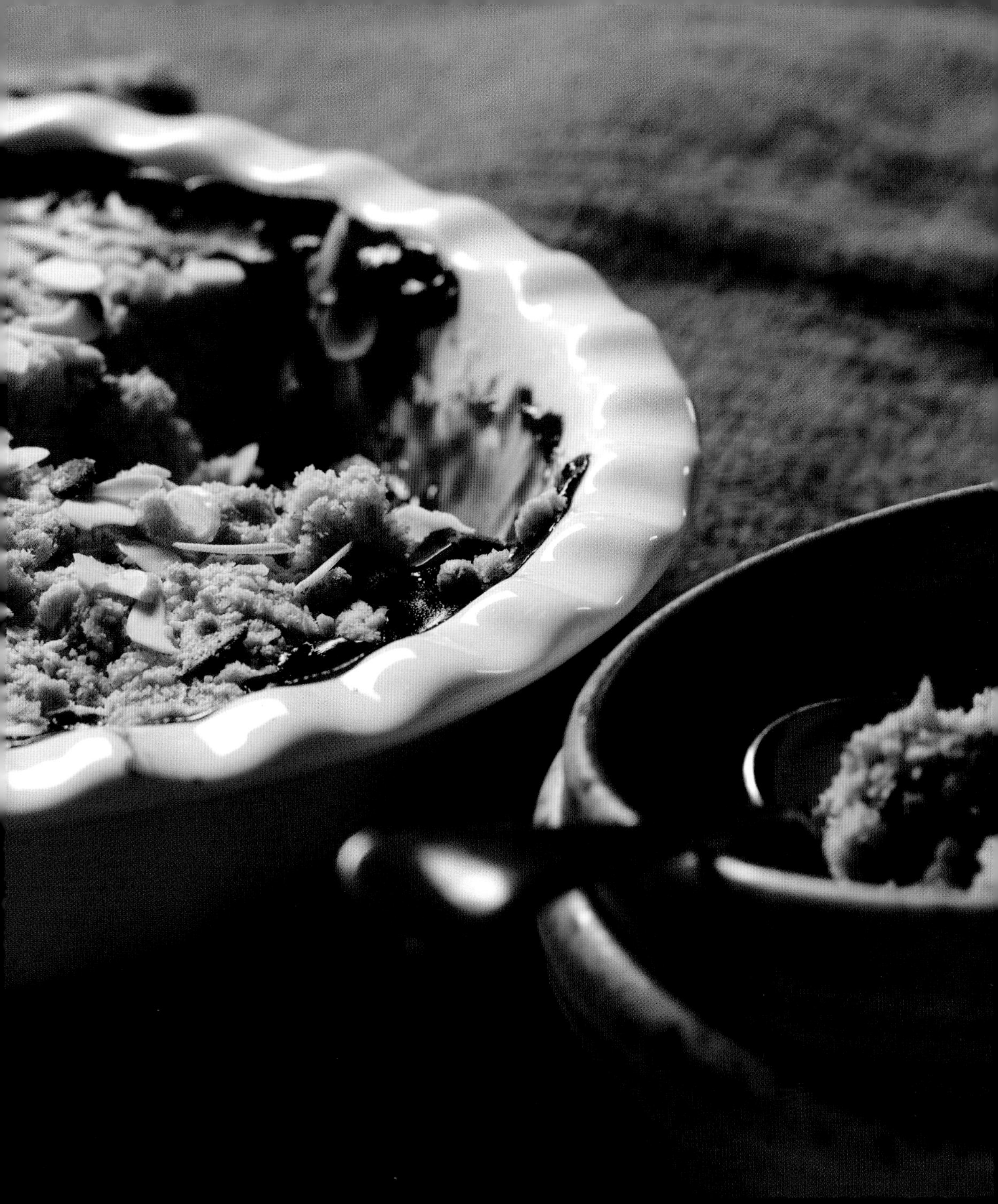

Banana, oat, sesame seed and walnut muffins

MAKES 12 MUFFINS
PREP: 15 minutes
COOK: 20–25 minutes

100 g/3½ oz porridge oats
200 g/7oz plain flour
1½ tsp baking powder
1 tsp bicarbonate of soda
¼ tsp sea salt
100 g/3½ oz light brown sugar
4 large ripe bananas
1 large free-range egg, beaten
60 g/2 oz melted butter
100 g/3½ oz chopped walnuts
4 tbsp sesame seeds
Demerara sugar, for sprinkling

These muffins are perfect to have around when you're feeling peckish in the evening – healthier and more sleep enhancing than a chocolate bar or potato chips. Walnuts contain their own melatonin and the oats provide the healthy carbs you need to absorb tryptophan speedily.

Preheat the oven to 180°C/350°F/gas mark 4. Line a 12-hole muffin tin with paper cases.

In a large bowl, combine the oats, flour, baking powder, bicarbonate of soda, sea salt and light brown sugar. Mix well and make a well in the centre of the mixture.

Mash the bananas with a fork in another bowl and stir in the beaten egg and melted butter.

Add to the dry mixture with the walnuts and sesame seeds, folding through gently until just combined – don't over-mix. Spoon into the paper cases and sprinkle with Demerara sugar.

Bake in the preheated oven for 20–25 minutes until golden brown and a skewer inserted into the middle of a muffin comes out clean.

Leave to cool and then store in an airtight container for up to five days.

Or you can try this ...

★ Use chopped pecans or hazelnuts.
★ Add some raisins or dried cherries to the mix.
★ Substitute light olive or sunflower oil for the butter.

Choc chip and hazelnut cookies

A cookie goes well with a hot milky drink at bedtime. White chocolate is lower in caffeine than dark chocolate and unlike other chocolate does not contain a stimulant called theobromine, which can increase heart rate and cause sleeplessness.

MAKES 20 COOKIES
PREP: 15 minutes
CHILL: 30 minutes
COOK: 20–25 minutes

120 g/4 oz hazelnuts
120 g/4 oz butter at room temperature
120 g/4 oz light brown sugar
1 large free-range egg, beaten
a few drops of vanilla extract
200 g/7 oz plain flour
175g/6oz white chocolate chips

Preheat the oven to 200°C/400°F/gas mark 6. Line two baking sheets with baking parchment.

Spread all the hazelnuts out on an unlined baking sheet and cook in the preheated oven for 4–5 minutes until toasted and lightly coloured. Allow to cool slightly and then put three-quarters of them in a processor. Blitz until coarsely ground. Cut the remaining nuts in half.

Reduce the oven temperature to 180°C/350°F/gas mark 4.

Beat the butter and sugar together until light and fluffy. You can use a hand-held electric whisk or a food mixer. Gradually beat in the egg, a little at a time, and then add the vanilla, flour, ground hazelnuts, chocolate chips and the halved hazelnuts. Mix to the consistency of a soft dough.

Put the dough on a clean work surface and roll into a long 7.5 cm/3 in thick sausage. Cover in cling film, twisting the ends, and chill in the fridge for at least 30 minutes to firm up.

Peel off the cling film and slice the dough into 20 discs. Arrange on the lined baking sheets and bake in the oven for 15–20 minutes until cooked and golden.

Cool on a wire rack and store in a tin, jar or other airtight container for up to five days.

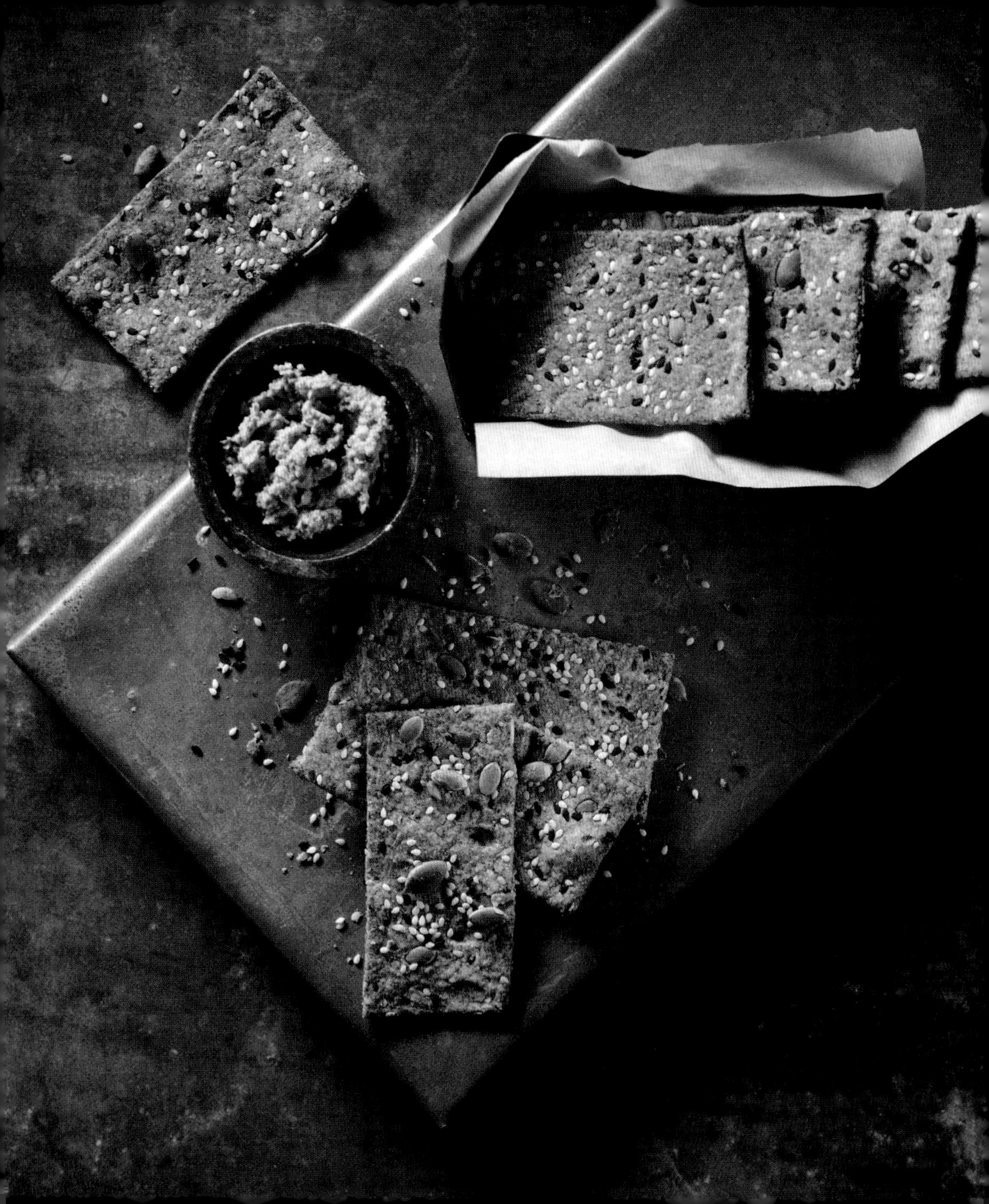

Seedy crisp cracker thins

Nibble these crisp crackers with some tangy cheese, hummus (see page 110) or tzatziki, which all contain tryptophan, when you fancy an evening snack. These healthy carbs will help speed up its absorption into your bloodstream.

MAKES 12 CRACKERS
PREP: 15 minutes
COOK: 10–12 minutes

150 g/5 oz rye flour
100 g/3½ oz wholemeal flour, plus extra for dusting
½ tsp baking powder
1 tsp fine sea salt
5 tbsp olive oil
150 ml/¼ pint water
85 g/3 oz pumpkin and black or white sesame seeds

Preheat the oven to 200°C/400°F/gas mark 6. Heat some non-stick baking sheets in the preheated oven.

Put the flours, baking powder and salt in a large mixing bowl. Make a well in the centre and pour in four tablespoons of olive oil and the water, drawing the flour in from the sides. Mix to a soft dough. If it's too sticky, add a little more flour; if it's too dry, add more water.

Knead the dough with your hands on a lightly floured surface until smooth. Roll out thinly as possible with a rolling pin, brush with the remaining olive oil and sprinkle with the seeds. Fold the dough over and roll the seeds into it. Knead lightly and divide into 12 pieces. Roll out each one really thinly.

Remove the hot baking sheets from the oven and carefully arrange the seeded dough thins on them. Bake in batches in the preheated oven for 10–12 minutes until crisp and golden.

Cool on a wire rack and store in a tin or other airtight container for up to five days.

Or you can try this ...

★ Use some caraway, fennel, cumin, chia or poppy seeds.
★ Sprinkle lightly with sea salt crystals before baking.

Greek honey roasted figs

SERVES 4
PREP: 10 minutes
COOK: 15 minutes

8 fresh ripe figs
grated zest and juice of 1 large juicy orange
3 tbsp clear Geek honey (thyme honey is best)
4 whole cloves
15 g/½ oz (1 tbsp) butter
240 g/8 oz 0% fat Greek yoghurt or katiki (Greek ewes' or goats' soft cheese)
60 g/2 oz chopped pistachio or hazelnuts

Figs contain sleep-enhancing potassium, calcium and magnesium and are one of the most delicious summer fruits. Because they're high in fibre they make us feel full, so we're less likely to experience hunger during the night.

Preheat the oven to 200°C/400°F/gas mark 6.

Cut a cross on the top of each fig and gently squeeze on the sides to open them. Arrange the figs in a large baking dish and pour the orange juice over them. Drizzle with two tablespoons of honey, add the cloves to the juice surrounding the figs and dot with the butter.

Bake in the preheated oven for 15 minutes until the figs are tender. Remove and set aside to cool. Discard the cloves.

In a bowl, mix together the yoghurt or katiki with the orange zest. Drizzle the remaining honey over the top.

Eat the figs warm or cold in their syrup, sprinkled with the nuts and served with the yoghurt or katiki.

Or you can try this…

★ Use lemon zest instead of orange.
★ Add a pinch of ground cinnamon to the orange juice and honey.
★ Stir some mascarpone or ricotta into the yoghurt.

Chocolate, orange and Greek yoghurt mousse

This healthy mousse is very light because it doesn't contain either cream or eggs. The high magnesium content of plain chocolate makes it a good choice for an evening dessert, especially when combined with milk and yoghurt.

SERVES 4
PREP: 10 minutes
COOK: 4–5 minutes
CHILL: 3 hours

250 g/9 oz plain chocolate (70% cocoa solids), coarsely chopped
240 ml/8 fl oz milk
3–4 tbsp caster sugar
grated zest of 1 orange
480 g/16 oz full-fat Greek yoghurt
grated chocolate or candied orange peel to serve

Put the chocolate, milk and sugar in a basin set over a pan of gently simmering water. Stir gently until the chocolate melts, the sugar dissolves and the mixture is smooth. Stir in the orange zest.

Beat the Greek yoghurt with a balloon whisk until light and fluffy.

Pour the melted chocolate over the yoghurt and fold in gently with a metal spoon in a figure-of-eight motion until well-mixed and evenly coloured.

Divide the mousse mixture between four small bowls and chill in the fridge for 3 hours minimum until set.

Serve sprinkled with grated chocolate or candied orange peel.

Or you can try this ...

★ Add a few drops of vanilla extract.
★ Sprinkle with cardamom seeds before serving.
★ Use slivers of orange zest instead of candied peel.

Chocolate rice pudding

SERVES 4
PREP: 5 minutes
COOK: 2 hours

85 g/3 oz short-grain pudding rice (dry weight)
2 tbsp caster sugar
600 ml/1 pint full-fat, semi-skimmed milk or almond milk
175 g/6 oz plain chocolate chips
1 vanilla pod, split lengthwise with seeds
15 g/½ oz butter, cut into tiny pieces, plus extra for greasing

This is one of the easiest and most delicious desserts you can make. The combination of milk and rice acts as a natural sedative. Plain chocolate is a good source of magnesium, which steadies heart rhythm and calms muscle and nerve function.

Preheat the oven to 150°C/300°F/gas mark 2. Generously butter a 1.2 litre/2 pint ovenproof dish.

Put the rice and sugar in the dish and pour in the milk. Stir to combine and then stir in the chocolate chips. Add the vanilla pod and seeds. Dot the top with butter.

Bake in the preheated oven for 2 hours until the rice is tender, the pudding is thick and creamy and there's a glossy brown skin on top. Check it after about 90 minutes and if it's too thick you can add a little milk.

Remove the vanilla pod and serve immediately.

Or you can try this…

★ Instead of a vanilla pod add a cinnamon stick.
★ Add the grated zest of an orange.
★ Use risotto rice if you don't have any pudding rice.

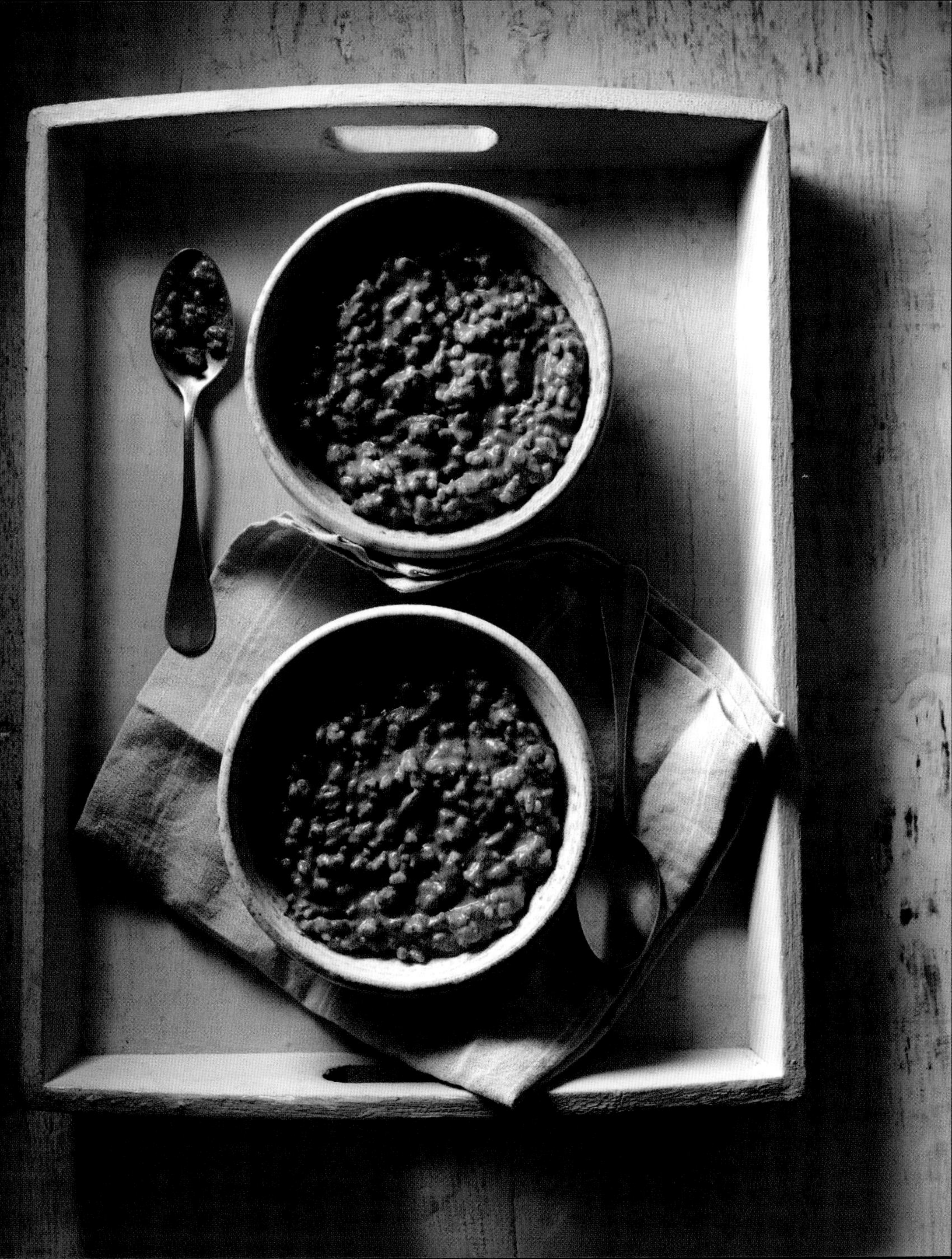

4

BEDTIME SNACKS

Chicken and mushroom broth

SERVES 4–6
PREP: 15 minutes
COOK: 20 minutes

2 tbsp olive oil
8 spring onions, sliced
1 garlic clove, crushed
1 tbsp finely chopped fresh root ginger
200 g/7 oz skinned chicken breast fillets, thinly sliced
100 g/3½ oz shiitake mushrooms, sliced
1.2 litres/2 pints fresh hot chicken stock
200 g/7 oz spring greens or spinach, shredded
100 g/3½ oz bean sprouts
1–2 tbsp dark soy sauce
a handful of fresh coriander, chopped

This soup is very light and a pre-bedtime bowl will provide vitamins B6 and D as well as tryptophan to ease you into a good night's sleep. If possible, use homemade fresh chicken stock for the best flavour and maximum nutritional benefit.

Heat the oil in a large saucepan set over a medium heat. When it's hot, add the spring onions, garlic, ginger, chicken and mushrooms. Cook for 5 minutes, stirring occasionally, until the vegetables are starting to soften and the chicken is golden brown.

Add the hot chicken stock and bring to the boil. Reduce the heat and simmer gently for 10 minutes.

Add the spring greens or spinach and cook gently for 5 minutes or until the chicken is cooked right through. Stir in the bean sprouts and soy sauce to taste.

Ladle the hot soup into bowls and serve piping hot sprinkled with coriander.

Or you can try this ...

★ Add a dash of lemon or lime juice or a spoonful of rice vinegar for a 'hot and sour' soup.
★ Add a lemongrass stalk and nam pla (Thai fish sauce) instead of soy sauce.
★ Add some thin carrot matchsticks.

Miso broth with seaweed and tofu

This is really quick and easy to prepare for a wholesome late-evening snack. Seaweed is a good source of calcium and magnesium, while the tofu contains calcium, potassium, magnesium and tryptophan.

SERVES 4–6
PREP: 5 minutes
STAND: 10–15 minutes
COOK: 12 minutes

1 tbsp dried wakame seaweed
1.2 litres/2 pints fresh vegetable stock
4 tbsp white miso paste
a small bunch of spring onions, finely sliced
200 g/7 oz thin asparagus, sliced
1 pak choi, trimmed and leaves separated
175 g/6 oz silken tofu, drained and cubed

Put the wakame in a bowl and cover with plenty of cold water. Set aside for 10–15 minutes until soft and rehydrated. Drain well.

Bring the stock to the boil in a large saucepan. Reduce the heat to a simmer and stir in the miso paste. Keep stirring until it dissolves.

Add the spring onions and asparagus and simmer gently for 3–4 minutes.

Stir in the pak choi and cook for 2 minutes, then add the tofu and wakame. Heat gently for 1–2 minutes.

Ladle the soup into bowls and serve piping hot.

Or you can try this …

- ★ Add some shredded greens, sliced enoki mushrooms or carrot cut into matchsticks.
- ★ Drizzle in a beaten egg at the end and stir with a fork to form long strands – it will take about 2 minutes.
- ★ Add some thin noodles.

Crispy kale chips

SERVES 4
PREP: 10 minutes
COOK: 12–15 minutes

200 g/7oz curly kale
2 tbsp olive oil
1 tsp paprika
sea salt flakes

Kale chips are a really healthy alternative to potato chips and they're delicious too. Eating plenty of dark leafy greens will give you the vitamins and minerals your body needs to support quality sleep.

Preheat the oven to 150°C/300°F/gas mark 2. Line two baking sheets with baking parchment.

Wash and dry the kale thoroughly – use a salad spinner or pat with a tea towel. Cut out and discard the thick central stems then tear the leaves into large bite-sized pieces.

Put the olive oil and paprika in a large bowl and add the kale, tossing it gently until coated all over with oil. Spread the pieces out in a single layer on the prepared baking sheets.

Bake in the preheated oven for about 15–20 minutes until crisp but still green. Sprinkle with sea salt flakes and leave to cool. They will crisp up even more. Eat within a day as they tend to lose their crispness and become soggy with time.

Or you can try this...

* Instead of regular paprika use the smoked variety or some ras-el-hanout.
* Add some ground toasted cumin seeds and grated lemon zest to the kale before cooking.
* Sprinkle a little grated cheese, e.g. Parmesan or Cheddar, over the kale towards the end of the cooking time.

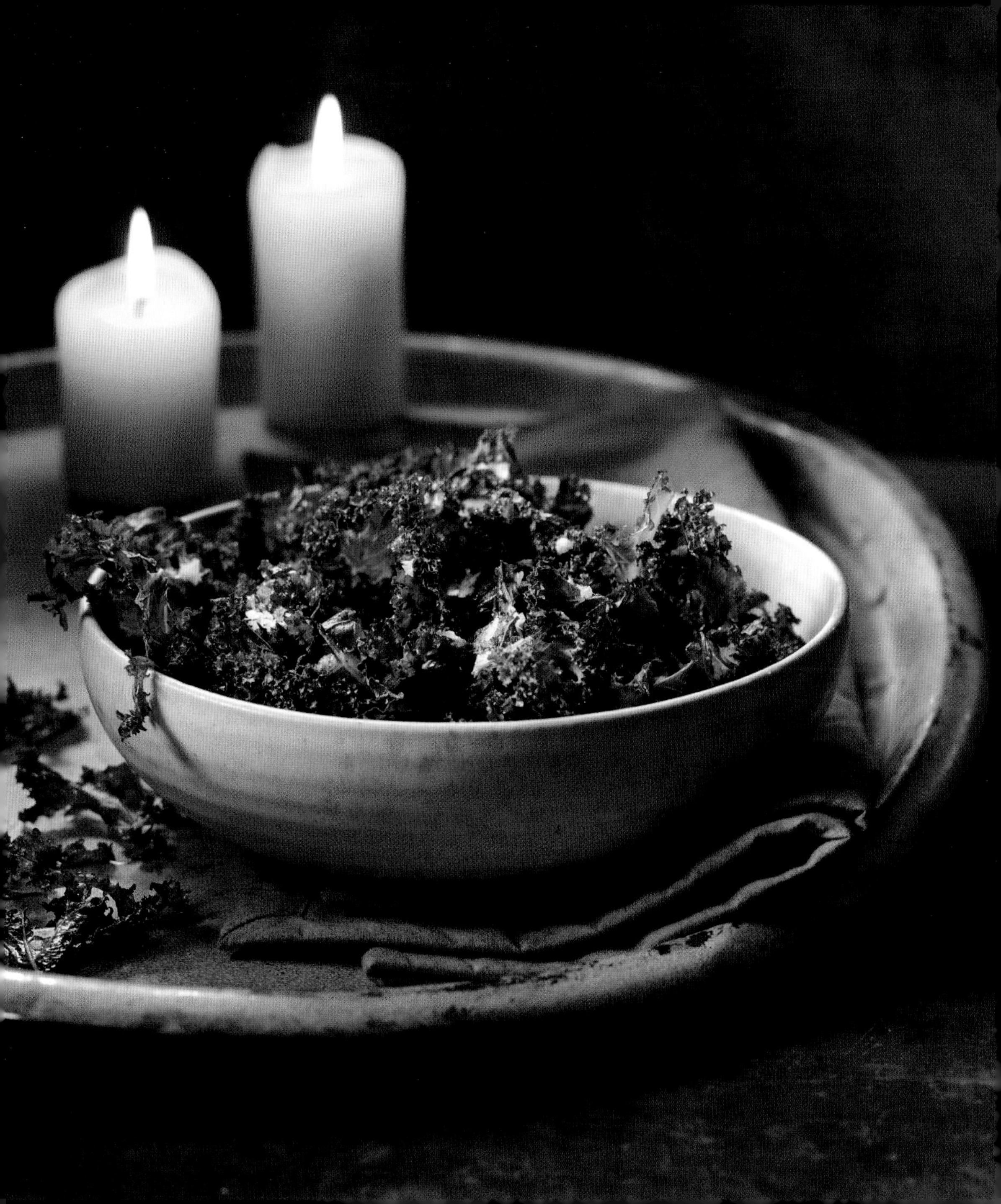

Green basil hummus with oatcakes

SERVES 4–6
PREP: 15 minutes

2 x 400 g/14 oz cans chickpeas
4 tbsp tahini
3–4 garlic cloves, crushed
½ tsp ground cumin
1 bunch fresh basil
1–2 tbsp olive oil, plus extra for drizzling
juice of 1 large lemon, plus extra for drizzling
a pinch of sea salt crystals
cumin seeds for sprinkling
oatcakes to serve

Hummus is quick and easy to make and it will keep well in the fridge for a few days. It's a good source of vitamin B6, as well as tryptophan. Eating hummus with oatcakes speeds up tryptophan absorption in the brain, shortening the time it takes to fall asleep.

Drain the chickpeas, reserving some of the liquid, and rinse under running cold water. Pat dry with kitchen paper.

Put most of the chickpeas (reserve a few for the garnish) in a blender or food processor with the tahini, garlic, cumin, basil, olive oil and lemon juice. Blitz to a coarse purée.

Add some of the reserved chickpea liquid or some extra olive oil or lemon juice until you end up with the consistency you want. The hummus should be quite soft (but not runny) and a little grainy, not too smooth. Season to taste with salt.

Transfer to a bowl and drizzle with olive oil and more lemon juice. Scatter with cumin seeds and the reserved whole chickpeas and serve with oatcakes.

Or you can try this…

★ Use fresh flat-leaf parsley, mint or coriander instead of basil.
★ Sprinkle with toasted seeds, e.g. pumpkin, sunflower, fennel or crushed coriander.
★ Make the texture more creamy by stirring in some 0% fat Greek yoghurt.

Wholemeal cheese straws with sesame seeds

Cheese straws are so delicious and good to munch if you feel hungry before going to bed. Wholemeal flour helps promote deep, restful sleep unlike white flour and other refined carbohydrates, which tend to reduce serotonin levels.

MAKES 25–30 CHEESE STRAWS
PREP: 15 minutes
CHILL: 30 minutes
COOK: 15–20 minutes

225 g/8 oz wholemeal flour
150 g/5 oz butter, diced
100 g/3½ oz grated Parmesan cheese
a pinch of mustard powder
1 small free-range egg, beaten
2 tbsp sesame seeds

Preheat the oven to 200°C/400°F/gas mark 6.

Put the flour in a large mixing bowl and rub in the butter with your fingertips until the mixture resembles coarse breadcrumbs. Stir in three-quarters of the grated cheese and the mustard powder. Mix in 1–2 tablespoons water – just enough to bring everything together and make a firm dough.

Place the dough in a plastic bag or wrap in some cling film and chill in the fridge for 30 minutes to firm it up.

Roll out the dough on a lightly floured surface until it's 5 mm/¼ in thick. Cut into thin strips and place on a lightly greased non-stick baking sheet. Brush with beaten egg and sprinkle with the sesame seeds and the remaining grated cheese.

Bake in the preheated oven for 15–20 minutes until crisp and golden. Leave to cool before storing in an airtight container. They will keep well for up to 1 week.

Or you can try this …

- ★ Sprinkle with poppy, caraway or cumin seeds.
- ★ Dust the cooked cheese straws with paprika.
- ★ Dip the cheese straws into some basil hummus (see opposite).

Moroccan roasted chickpeas

MAKES 500 G/1LB 2OZ
PREP: 10 minutes
COOK: 25–35 minutes

2 x 400 g/14 oz cans chickpeas, drained and rinsed
2 tbsp olive oil
½ tsp fine sea salt
1 tsp cumin seeds, coarsely ground
½ tsp ground coriander seeds, coarsely ground
½ tsp ground cinnamon
¼ tsp ground ginger
½ tsp paprika
¼ tsp light brown sugar

The gently spicy cumin and coriander seeds and ginger boost the mineral content, as well as aiding digestion. They have been used as a natural remedy for insomnia since ancient times.

Preheat the oven to 200°C/400°F/gas mark 6.

Put the chickpeas in a bowl with the olive oil and sea salt, seeds, ground spices, paprika and sugar. Toss lightly together until they are evenly coated.

Spread the chickpeas out in a single layer on a baking sheet with a raised edge. Roast in the preheated oven for 25–35 minutes, turning once or twice, until crisp and golden brown. Check towards the end of the cooking time to make sure they don't burn.

Remove from the oven and leave to cool on the tray. Store in a sealed container or plastic bag at room temperature. They will stay crisp and fresh for a few days.

Or you can try this…

* Add some ground allspice or cloves.
* Add some herbs, e.g. oregano or basil.
* Stir in some grated lemon zest.

Salted edamame beans

You don't have to go to your local Japanese restaurant to enjoy eating salted edamame – you can make them yourself at home. Researchers in Japan have discovered that people who eat soybeans regularly tend to sleep soundly.

SERVES 4
PREP: 5 minutes
COOK: 5 minutes

450 g / 1 lb fresh or frozen edamame beans in their pods
sea salt flakes for sprinkling

If using fresh edamame beans, bring a large saucepan of water to a rolling boil and add some salt. Tip in the beans and boil for 5 minutes until tender. If using frozen, follow the instructions on the packet.

Drain well in a colander and pat dry with kitchen paper.

Transfer to a bowl and sprinkle with sea salt before serving. Only eat the tender beans, not the stringy pods.

Or you can try this …

- ★ Sprinkle the cooked beans with black and white sesame seeds.
- ★ Drizzle with sesame oil.
- ★ Toss the cooked beans with some crushed garlic that has been cooked in sesame oil for 1–2 minutes until tender but not coloured.

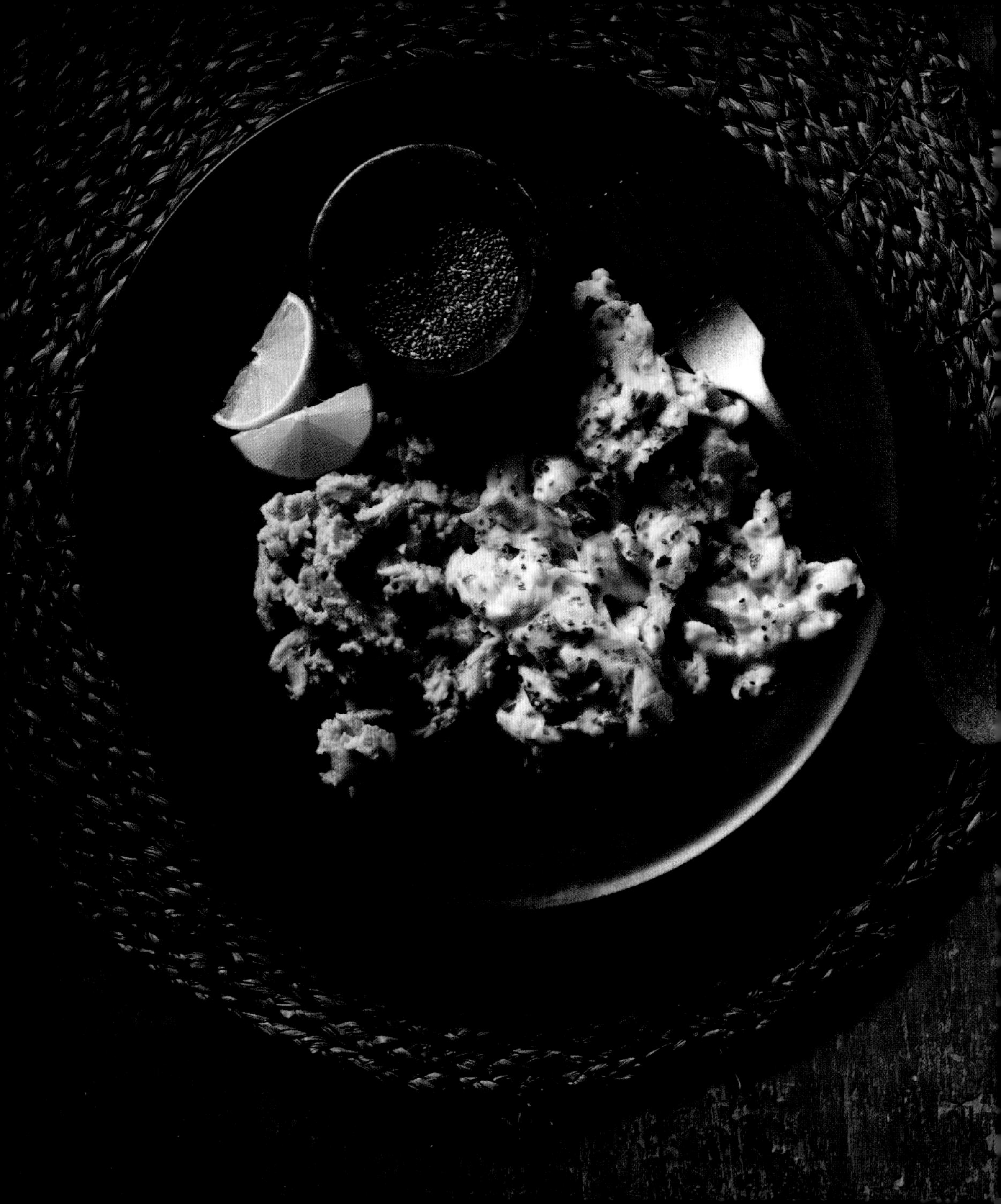

Chia seed scrambled eggs with avocado smash

Scrambled eggs make a comforting and nutritious bedtime snack, and they're so quick and easy to make. Eggs and milk contain the natural sedative tryptophan and are also a good source of vitamin D.

SERVES 2
PREP: 5 minutes
COOK: 5 minutes

1 ripe avocado, stoned and peeled
a squeeze of lime juice
4 medium free-range eggs
3 tbsp milk
1 tbsp chia seeds
a few fresh parsley sprigs, chopped
1 tbsp olive oil
15 g/½ oz (1 tbsp) butter
sea salt and freshly ground black pepper

Mash the avocado flesh roughly with a fork and stir in the lime juice. Season with sea salt and some black pepper.

Beat the eggs with the milk in a bowl. Add the chia seeds and parsley, and season lightly with salt and pepper.

Heat the oil and butter in a non-stick pan set over a low to medium heat. Pour in the egg mixture and stir with a wooden spoon until the eggs start to scramble and set. When they have thickened and there's no liquid left in the pan, remove from the heat.

Divide the scrambled eggs between two plates and eat immediately with the smashed avocado, lime wedges and extra chia seeds.

Or you can try this …

★ Add some chopped spring onions to the scrambled eggs.
★ Add some grated cheese to the scrambled eggs.
★ Serve rolled up in a warm tortilla or seedy wrap.

Smoked mackerel pâté

SERVES 4–6
PREP: 10 minutes

3 smoked mackerel fillets, skinned
120 g/4 oz cream cheese
100 g/3½ oz crème fraîche
grated zest and juice of ½ lemon
1–2 tsp creamed horseradish
a few fresh flat-leaved parsley sprigs, chopped
oatcakes or wholemeal crackers to serve

This is really quick and easy to make and it wil keep in the fridge for several days in a sealed container. Mackerel contains magnesium that will calm your body and mind for sleep.

Put all the ingredients in a blender or food processor and blitz until smooth.

Transfer to a bowl, cover and chill until required. Serve with oatcakes or wholemeal crackers.

Or you can try this...

★ Use dill or tarragon instead of parsley.
★ Add some capers or a small bunch of watercress.
★ Substitute a 200 g/7 oz can of salmon for the mackerel.

Smoked salmon pâté

Eating some wholemeal crackers or a couple of oatcakes topped with a little homemade fish pâté can relax you and help prevent nighttime hunger pangs and wakefulness.

SERVES 4
PREP: 10 minutes
CHILL: 1 hour

200 g/7 oz smoked salmon
100 g/3½ oz cream cheese
100 g/3½ oz 0% fat Greek yoghurt
1 tbsp mayonnaise
grated zest and juice of 1 small lemon
1 tsp chopped capers
a handful of fresh dill, chopped
oatcakes or wholemeal crackers to serve

Briefly blitz the salmon in a food processor or blender with the cream cheese, yoghurt, mayonnaise, lemon zest and juice.

Stir in the capers and herbs and transfer to a bowl. Cover and chill in the fridge for at least 1 hour.

Serve with oatcakes or wholemeal crackers.

Or you can try this …

★ Add a dash of creamed horseradish.
★ Stir in some finely chopped spring onions or chives.
★ Instead of smoked salmon, use a 200 g/7 oz can of drained tuna in spring water.
★ Substitute crème fraîche for Greek yoghurt.

Chia seed and banana porridge

SERVES 2
PREP: 10 minutes
COOK: 1–2 minutes
CHILL: 3 hours +

1 large banana, mashed
4 tbsp chia seeds
300 ml/½ pint unsweetened almond milk
a few drops of vanilla extract
2 tbsp Greek yoghurt
clear honey for drizzling

FOR THE TOASTED NUTS AND SEEDS:
2 tbsp chopped walnuts
2 tbsp flax, hemp or pumpkin seeds
2 tbsp dried cherries
1 tbsp coconut flakes

As well as being a great source of protein, chia seeds contain tryptophan, the amino acid that raises your melatonin and serotonin levels, making you feel relaxed and sleepy.

Put the banana and chia seeds in a bowl with the almond milk. Whisk until everything is combined and there are no big lumps of banana.

Leave to stand for 2–3 minutes, then whisk in the vanilla. The porridge should be starting to thicken already. Cover and chill in the fridge for several hours or overnight.

Toast the nuts and seeds: heat a small dry frying pan over a medium heat. Add the walnuts and seeds and heat, tossing them gently once or twice, for 1–2 minutes until golden. Make sure they don't burn. Remove and mix with the cherries and coconut flakes. Allow to cool.

When the banana and chia mixture has thickened to the consistency of tapioca-like porridge, divide it between two bowls and top with a spoonful of yoghurt. Sprinkle with the toasted nuts and seeds and drizzle with honey.

Or you can try this…

★ Use dried blueberries, cranberries or raisins.
★ Add some sunflower seeds.
★ Flavour with grated lemon or orange zest or a pinch of ground cinnamon.

Fresh figs dipped in dark chocolate and nuts

Figs are rich in magnesium – the mineral that improves the quality, length and restfulness of our sleep – as well as calcium, which helps the brain to make melatonin.

MAKES 12 FIGS
PREP: 15 minutes
SET: 30 minutes – 2 hours

175 g/6 oz plain chocolate (70% cocoa solids)
12 fresh figs
60 g/2 oz finely chopped walnuts

Chop the chocolate into pieces and place in a heatproof bowl suspended over a pan of simmering water. When the chocolate melts, remove from the heat. Alternatively, melt the chocolate in a microwave.

Take a fig and holding it by its stem, carefully dip the round end into the melted chocolate, coating it about halfway up. Shake off any excess.

Dip the chocolate-coated end into the chopped walnuts and place on a tray lined with greaseproof paper. Repeat with the remaining figs.

Leave in a cool place for about 2 hours until the chocolate sets hard, or chill in the fridge for 30 minutes. Store in a sealed container in the fridge.

Or you can try this ...

★ Use chopped hazelnuts, pecans, almonds or pistachios.
★ You can use plump dried figs instead of fresh ones.
★ Add some grated orange zest to the melted chocolate.
★ Drizzle a little honey over the figs before eating them.

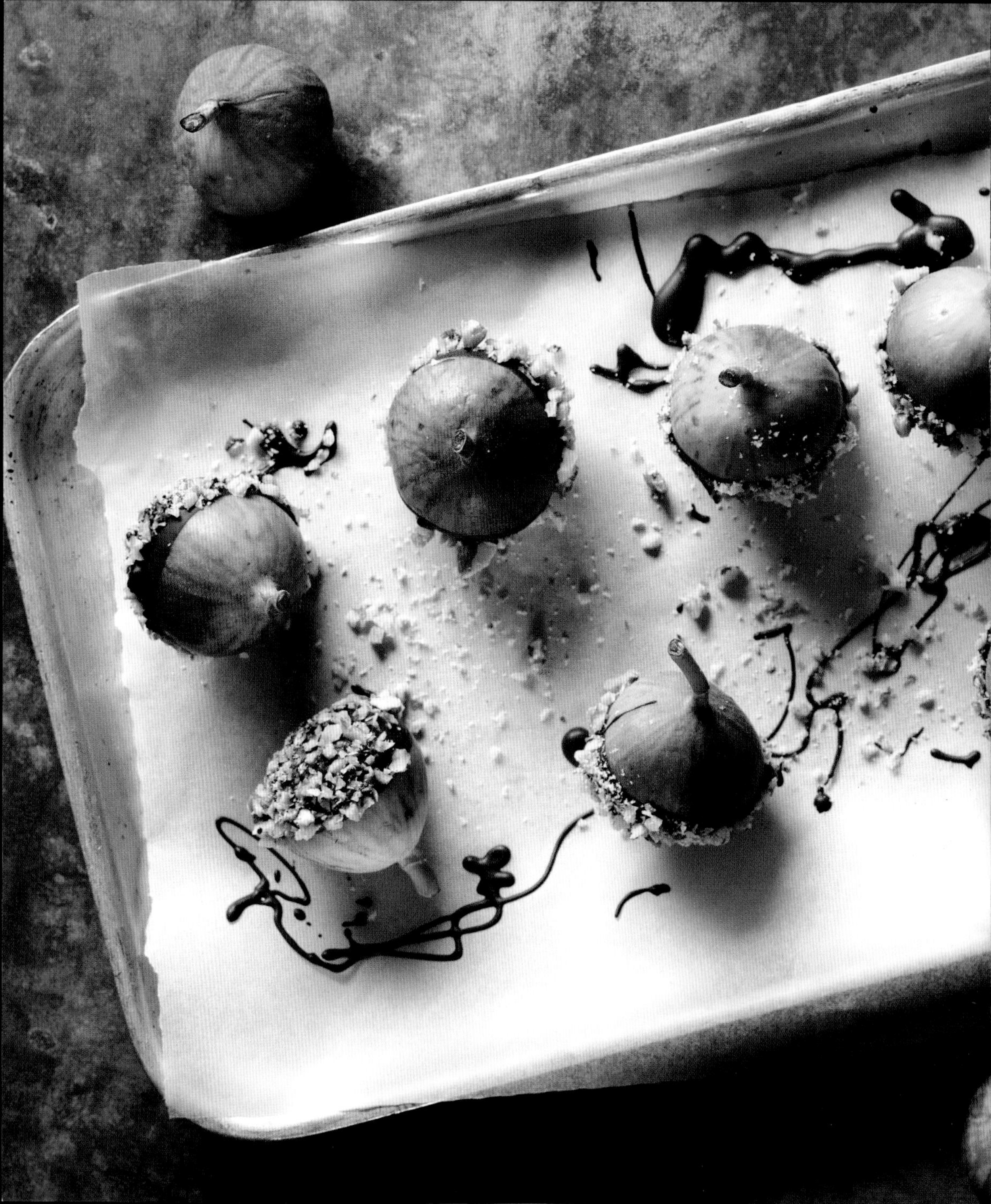

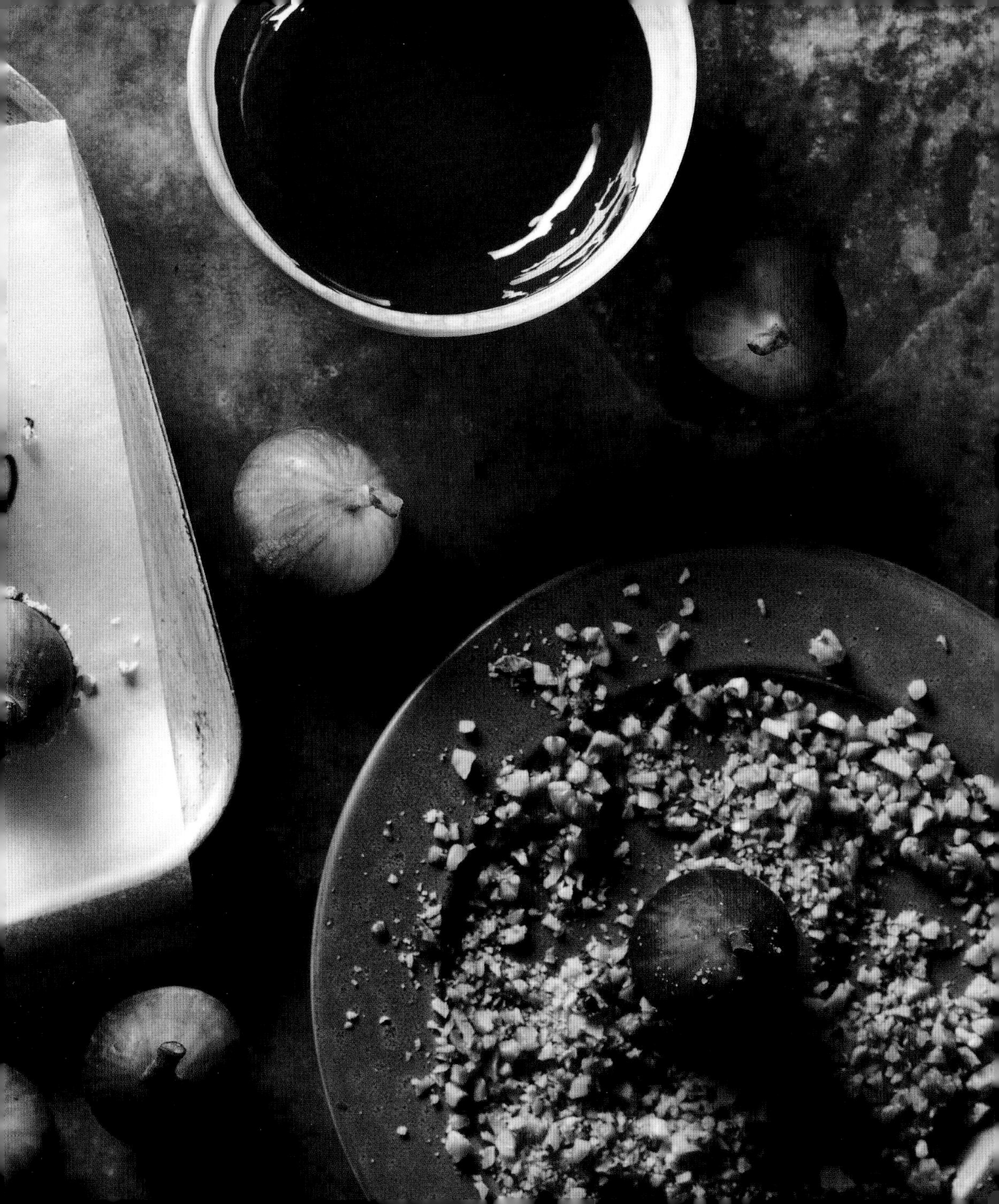

Fruity, nutty oat and yoghurt pots

SERVES 2
PREP: 10 minutes
CHILL: 4 hours +

240 g/8 oz 0% fat Greek yoghurt
a few drops of vanilla extract
60 ml/2 fl oz almond milk or soya milk
4 tbsp porridge oats
2 tbsp mixed seeds, e.g. pumpkin, sunflower, linseed, chia
2 tbsp chopped almonds
60 g/2 oz raisins or chopped dried figs, dates, apricots or prunes
1 banana, sliced
2 tsp clear honey

It's easy to make these little pots earlier in the day and then leave them to chill in the fridge for a few hours until the yoghurt and milk soften the oats. They combine all the sleep-friendly foods you need for relaxation and good digestion.

Mix most of the Greek yoghurt with the vanilla extract, milk, porridge oats, seeds and nuts.

Divide the mixture between four shallow glass jars or clear containers and cover with the dried fruit. Top with the remaining yoghurt.

Cover and leave in the fridge for at least 4 hours or even overnight. Serve topped with sliced banana, drizzled with honey.

Or you can try this …

★ Flavour the yoghurt with some grated orange zest.
★ Instead of banana, top with some papaya (pawpaw).
★ Substitute chopped walnuts, hazelnuts or pistachios for the almonds.

Nut butter toast with banana

These toasties are the nutritional equivalent of a sleeping pill and they contain all the sleep-friendly nutrients you need. Sometimes it's good to have a snack before bed, especially if it's several hours since you last ate.

SERVES 2
PREP: 5 minutes

2 slices wholemeal bread
3 tbsp almond or cashew butter
2 small ripe bananas

Toast the bread lightly and spread with the almond or cashew butter.

Peel the bananas and either mash them or slice them. Arrange on top of the toasties and eat immediately.

Or you can try this…

★ Use crunchy peanut butter (no added salt or sugar).
★ You could also add some sliced cherries, which are great for boosting melatonin.
★ Dust the banana with ground cinnamon.
★ Use four slices of toasted bread and sandwich together.

Seedy homemade granola bowl

SERVES 4
PREP: 10 minutes
COOK: 20–25 minutes

30 g/1 oz coconut oil
2 tbsp maple syrup
100 g/3½ oz rolled oats
4 tbsp roughly chopped walnuts
3 tbsp flaked almonds
25 g/1 oz sunflower seeds
25 g/1 oz pumpkin seeds
2 tbsp sesame seeds
4 tbsp raisins
a pinch of ground cinnamon

TO SERVE:
Greek or low-fat yoghurt
clear honey for drizzling
stoned fresh cherries

Granola makes a great bedtime snack as well as a breakfast cereal. Serve it with cherries, which boost your melatonin levels, and honey. The natural sugar in honey sends a message to the brain to stop producing orexin, a chemical that triggers alertness.

Preheat the oven to 160°C/325°F/gas mark 3.

Make the granola: heat the coconut oil and maple syrup in a pan set over a low heat until the coconut oil melts. Stir in the oats, walnuts, almonds, seeds, raisins and cinnamon – everything should be well coated.

Spread the mixture out in a thin layer on a large baking sheet. Bake in the preheated oven for 15–20 minutes, stirring once or twice, until golden brown and crisp. Leave to cool, then transfer to an airtight container.

Serve the granola with the yoghurt, drizzled with honey, and the cherries.

Or you can try this ...

★ Use flax, sesame and sunflower seeds.
★ Add some chopped dates or dried figs.
★ Instead of cherries, serve with sliced banana or papaya.

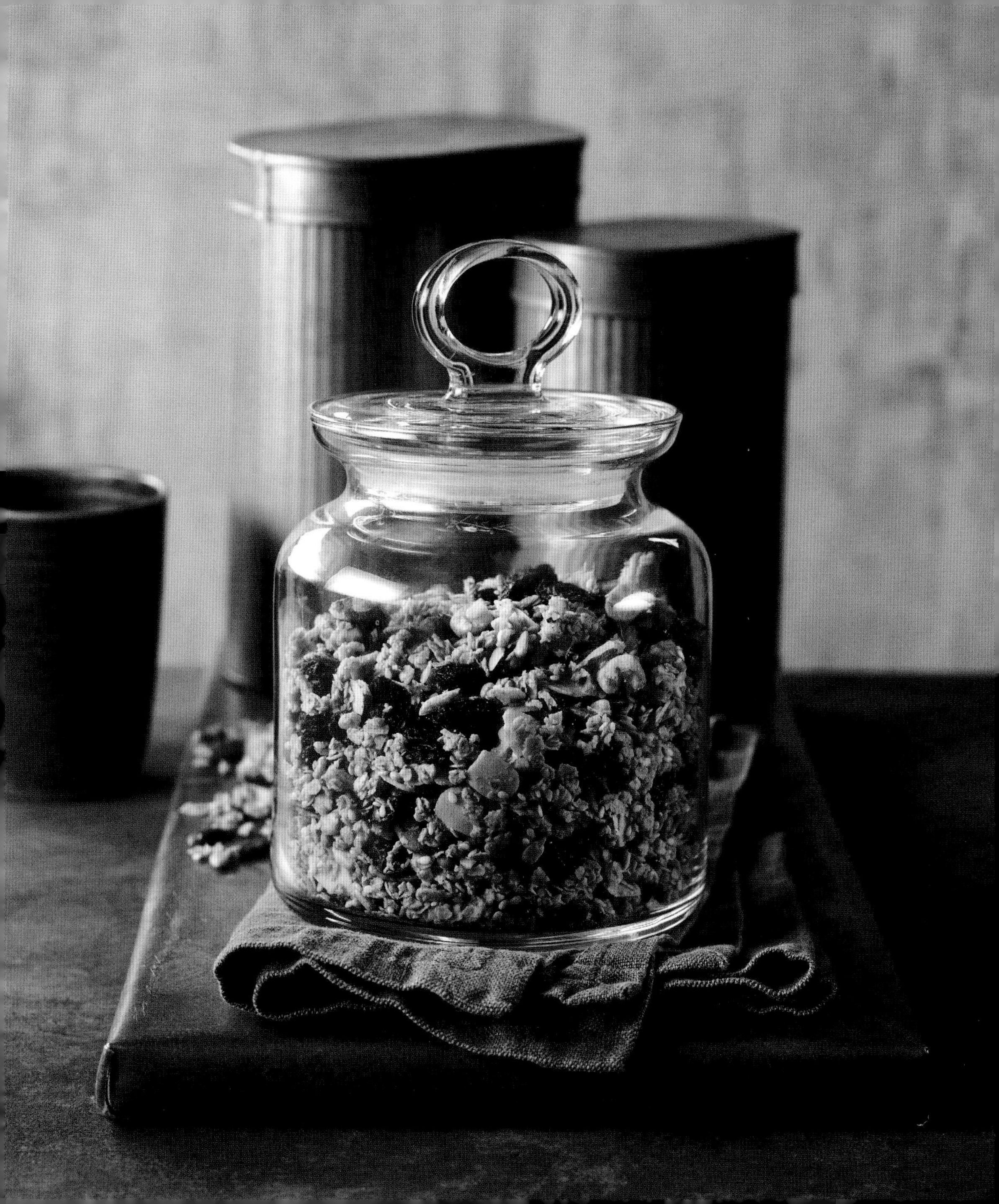

Oat porridge with chocolate and cherry compôte

SERVES 2
PREP: 5 minutes
COOK: 15–20 minutes

85 g/3 oz porridge oats
a pinch of salt
200 ml/7 fl oz almond or soya milk
200 ml/7 fl oz water
2 tbsp 0% fat Greek yoghurt
30 g/1 oz dark chocolate (70% cocoa solids), coarsely grated

FOR THE CHERRY COMPÔTE:
300 g/10 oz cherries, stoned
2 tbsp water
1 tbsp clear honey

Oats are comforting and rich in potassium, magnesium, calcium and tryptophan, all of which help to produce good quality sleep. Because they're low GI (glycaemic index) they release energy slowly to keep you sleeping soundly throughout the night.

Make the cherry compôte: put the cherries and water in a saucepan and poach gently over a low heat for 8–10 minutes until the cherries are tender but still hold their shape. Remove the cherries with a slotted spoon and add the honey to the juices in the pan. Turn up the heat and cook until reduced and thick enough to coat the back of a spoon. Pour over the cherries and set aside, or leave to cool, then cover and chill in the fridge until required.

Put the porridge oats, salt, milk and water in a non-stick pan and bring to the boil, stirring. Reduce the heat to a bare simmer and cook gently, stirring, until thickened, smooth and creamy.

Serve the porridge topped with the yoghurt and grated chocolate, and with the cherry compôte.

Or you can try this ...

★ Use frozen cherries instead of fresh ones.
★ Use regular milk instead of almond or soya.
★ Add some grated orange zest to the cherries.

Bedtime blitz

You'll need a food blender to make this surprisingly filling snack. Packed with sleep-friendly foods, it's full of natural goodness and very soothing, as well as being quick and easy to make.

SERVES 2
PREP: 10 minutes

1 large banana, peeled and cut into chunks
60 g/2 oz stoned cherries, hulled strawberries or papaya
30 g/1 oz stoned dates or prunes
85 g/3 oz raw broccoli florets
2 tbsp mixed seeds, e.g. pumpkin and sunflower
2 tsp chia seeds
2 tbsp ground linseed
1 tbsp cacao nibs
1 tsp ground turmeric
½ tsp freshly grated nutmeg
30 g/1 oz walnuts, almonds or hazelnuts
240 g/8 oz probiotic plain yoghurt
60 ml/2 fl oz fresh or unsweetened orange juice
almond milk or soya milk to thin to desired consistency

Put all the ingredients except the milk in a food processor or large blender and pulse until thoroughly combined and thick.

Add some almond or soya milk, a little at a time, and pulse until you have the desired consistency.

Pour into two glasses and enjoy!

Or you can try this …

★ Add some spirulina powder.
★ Add some raw spinach, kale or spring greens.
★ Add some flaxseeds, sesame seeds or hemp seeds.
★ Add some peeled fresh root ginger.
★ Flavour with a few drops of vanilla extract, some ground cinnamon or ground ginger.

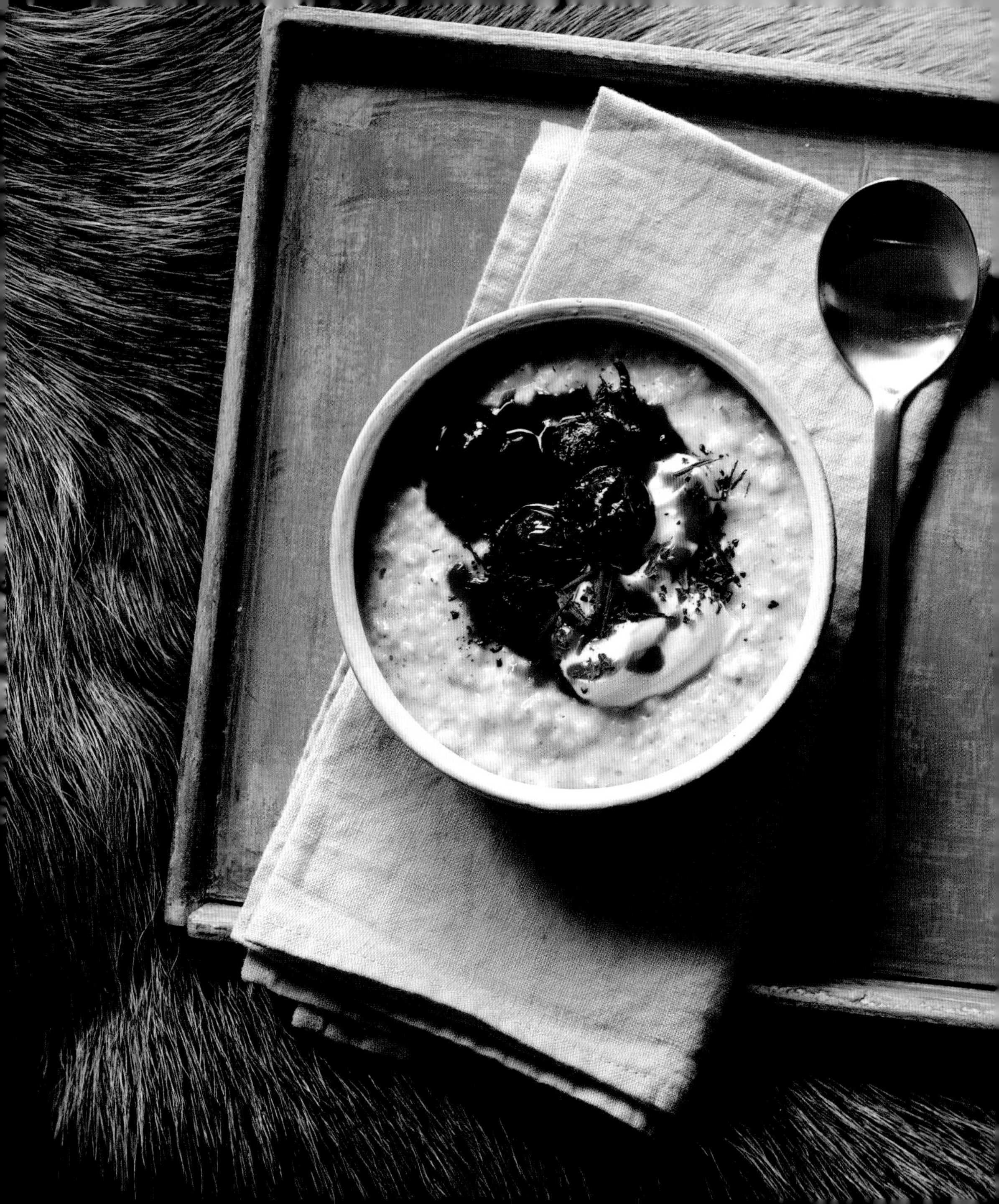

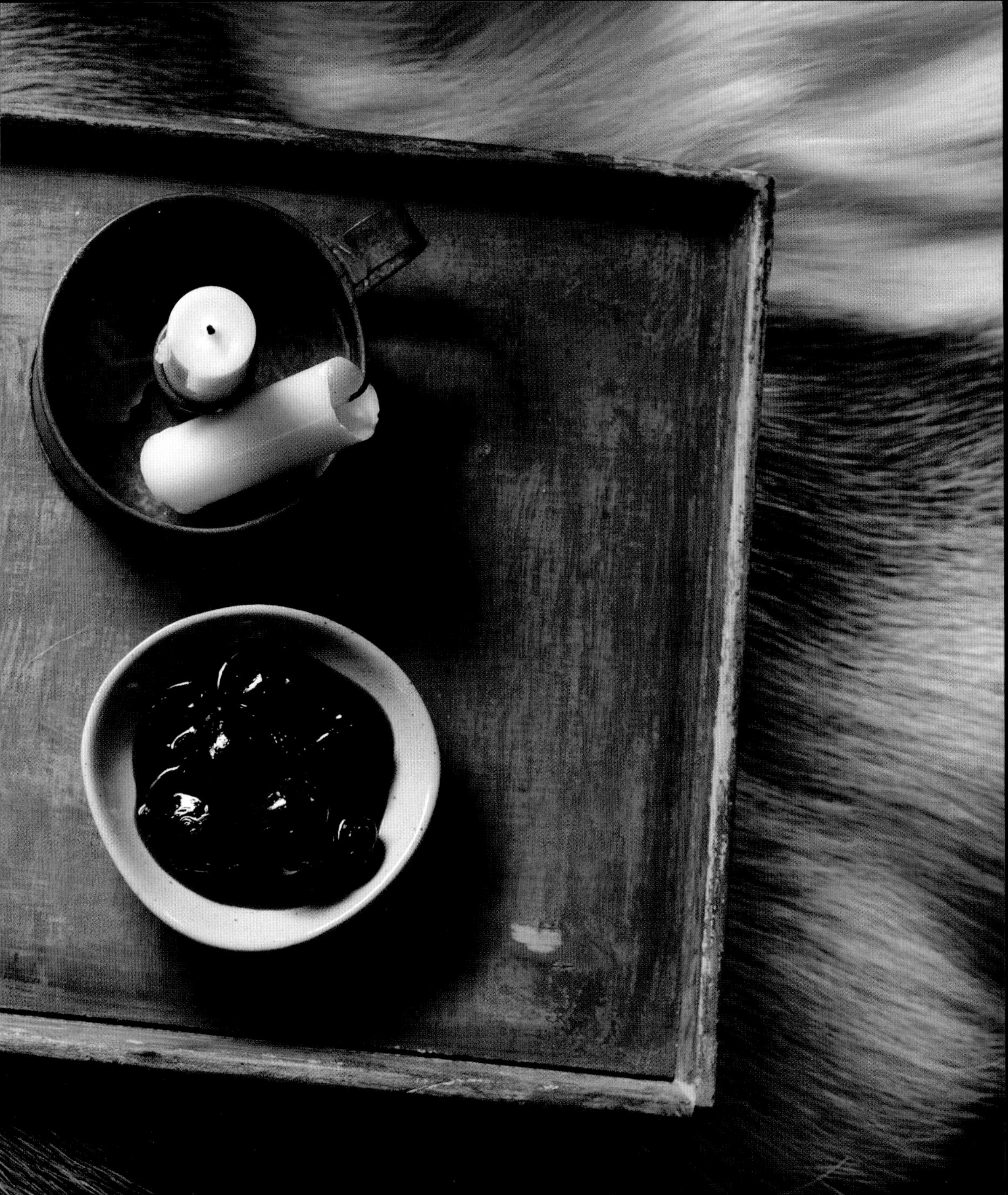

5

BEDTIME DRINKS

Kale and avocado smoothie

SERVES 2
PREP: 10 minutes

60 g/2 oz curly kale, stalks removed
½ cucumber
1 ripe avocado, stoned and peeled
a handful of fresh basil
1 large banana, fresh or frozen
1 tbsp flaxseeds
240 g/8 oz % fat Greek yoghurt
120 ml/4 fl oz almond milk

Smoothies are not just for breakfast – they make great bedtime drinks, too. Delicious and packed with nutrients, they're quick and easy to prepare and make you feel full.

Put all the ingredients in a blender and blitz until really smooth.

Pour the smoothie into two glasses and serve immediately.

Or you can try this…

★ Use pumpkin, sunflower or chia seeds, or a mixture of them all.
★ Add a dash of fresh lime juice or some peeled fresh root ginger.
★ Use probiotic natural yoghurt.
★ Add some walnuts or almonds, or even a handful of oats.
★ Sweeten with honey.

Peanut butter and banana smoothie

You probably know how well peanut butter and bananas go together but have you ever thought of combining them in a smoothie? Peanut butter is a great way to boost your magnesium levels – if they're low, it's harder to sleep.

SERVES 2
PREP: 5 minutes

2 tbsp unsweetened peanut butter
1 large banana
120 g/4 oz 0% fat Greek yoghurt
300 ml/½ pint almond milk
a few drops of vanilla extract

Put all the ingredients in a blender and blitz until smooth.

Pour into two glasses and serve immediately.

Or you can try this…

★ Use soya milk or regular full-fat or semi-skimmed milk.
★ Substitute one tablespoon of tahini for the peanut butter.
★ Sweeten to taste with clear honey.
★ Add a handful of oats.

Papaya and chia seed smoothie

SERVES 2
PREP: 10 minutes

1 papaya
1 large banana
180 ml/6 fl oz soya milk
180 g/6 oz probiotic natural yoghurt
a few drops of vanilla extract
1 tbsp chia seeds

This simple smoothie contains the essential nutrients you need to promote a good night's sleep. Papayas are a good source of magnesium, potassium and calcium which help to regulate our metabolism and prevent insomnia.

Cut the papaya in half and discard the seeds. Scoop out the flesh and put in a blender with the rest of the ingredients.

Blitz all the ingredients in the blender until really smooth and creamy. If the smoothie is too thick for your liking, add some more soya milk.

Pour into two glasses and serve immediately, with ice if wished.

Or you can try this…

★ Add some walnuts, pecans or hazelnuts.
★ Add one or two tablespoons of wheatgerm.
★ Add two tablespoons of muesli.
★ Sweeten with some clear honey.

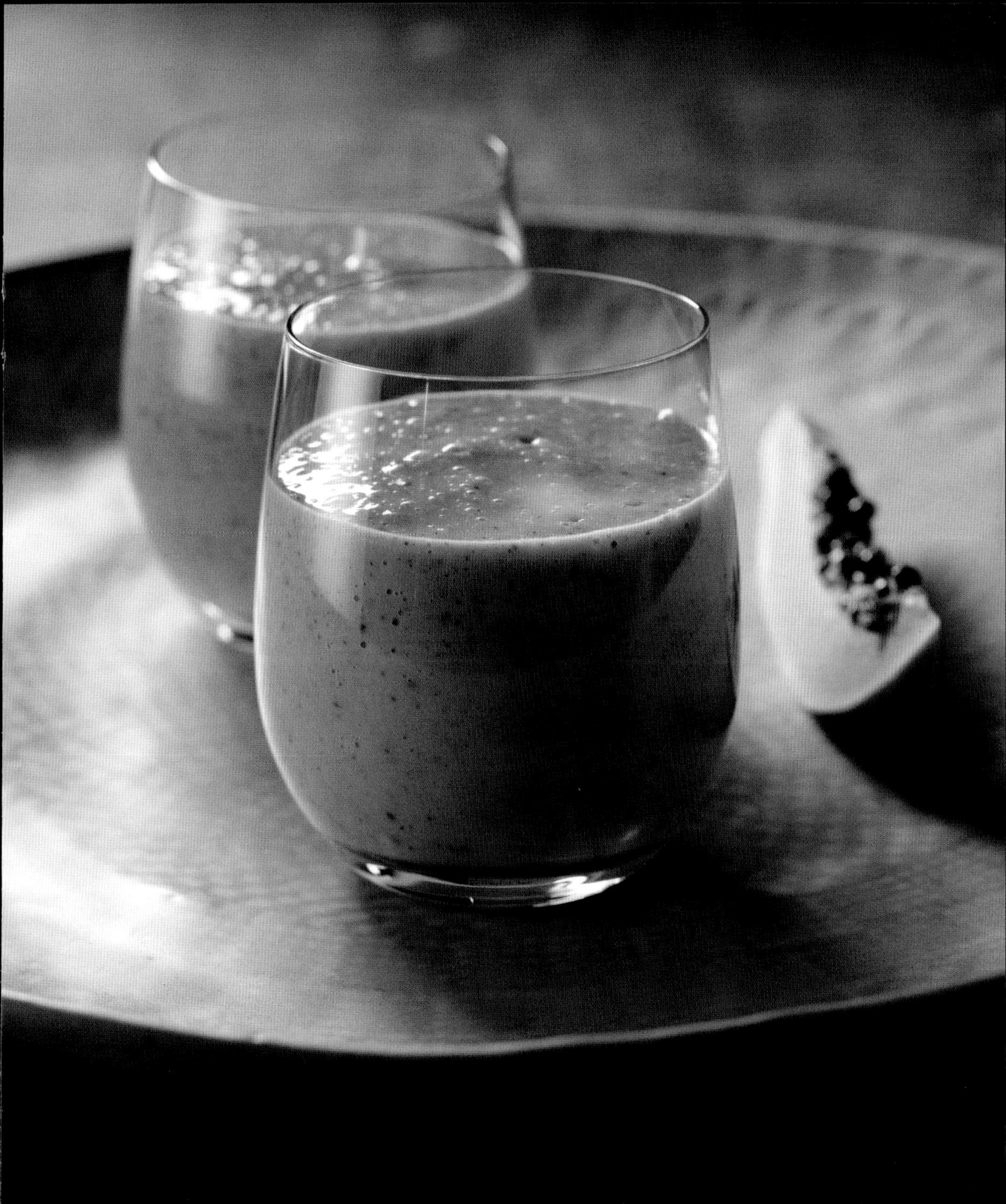

Soya and cherry smoothie

SERVES 2
PREP: 5 minutes

225 g/8 oz fresh cherries, stoned
1 ripe banana
240 ml/8 fl oz soya milk
120 g/4 oz probiotic yoghurt
1 tsp clear honey

This smoothie not only tastes good, it does you good. Soya milk contains the calming tryptophan and cherries boost melatonin; eating them regularly may help to relieve insomnia.

Put all the ingredients in a blender and blitz until smooth. If the smoothie is too thick for your liking, add some more soya milk.

Pour into two glasses and serve immediately.

Or you can try this …

- Use almond or cashew milk instead of soya.
- Use orange juice instead of yoghurt for a thinner smoothie.
- Add a kiwi fruit or some papaya (pawpaw).
- Add a dash of lemon or lime juice.

Hot chocolate drink with honey

Nothing beats a mug of hot chocolate made with the real stuff – not cocoa powder. Plain chocolate is a good source of magnesium, which helps us unwind and relaxes aching muscles, as well as reducing and regulating the body's levels of cortisol.

SERVES 2
PREP: 10 minutes

480 ml/16 fl oz almond or soya milk
85 g/3 oz plain chocolate (70% cocoa solids), chopped or grated
a pinch of ground cinnamon
clear honey to taste

Pour one-third of the milk into a saucepan and set over a medium heat. Add the chocolate and stir until it melts into the milk.

Add the remaining milk and the cinnamon and whisk into the chocolate milk.

When the milk is really hot, remove from the heat before it boils and give it a good whisk until it's frothy.

Pour into two mugs and serve immediately, sweetened with honey to taste.

Or you can try this ...

★ Dust with cinnamon rather than stirring it into the hot milk.
★ Top with freshly grated nutmeg.
★ Add some ground cardamom.
★ Add some vanilla seeds or extract.

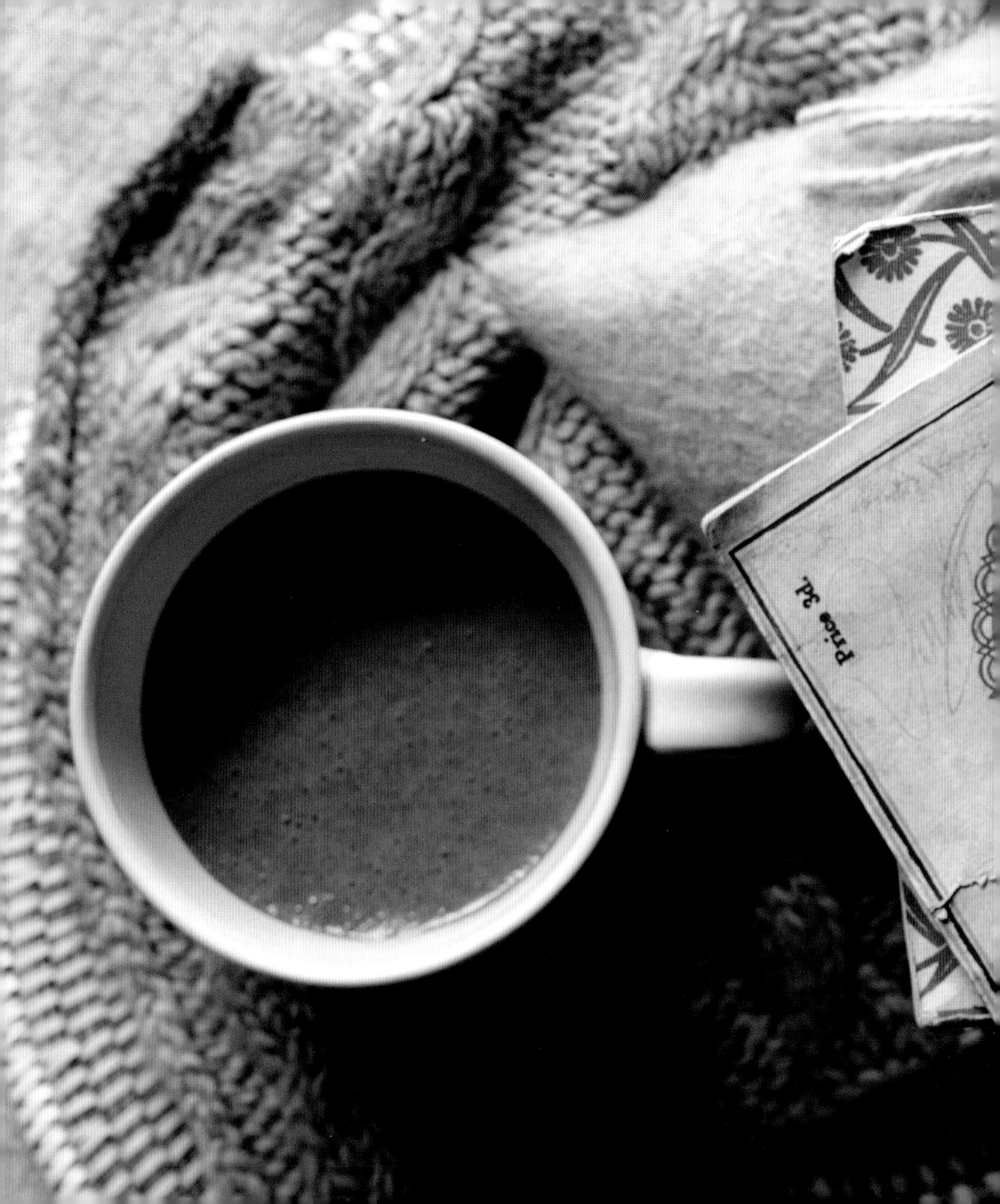
Price 3d.

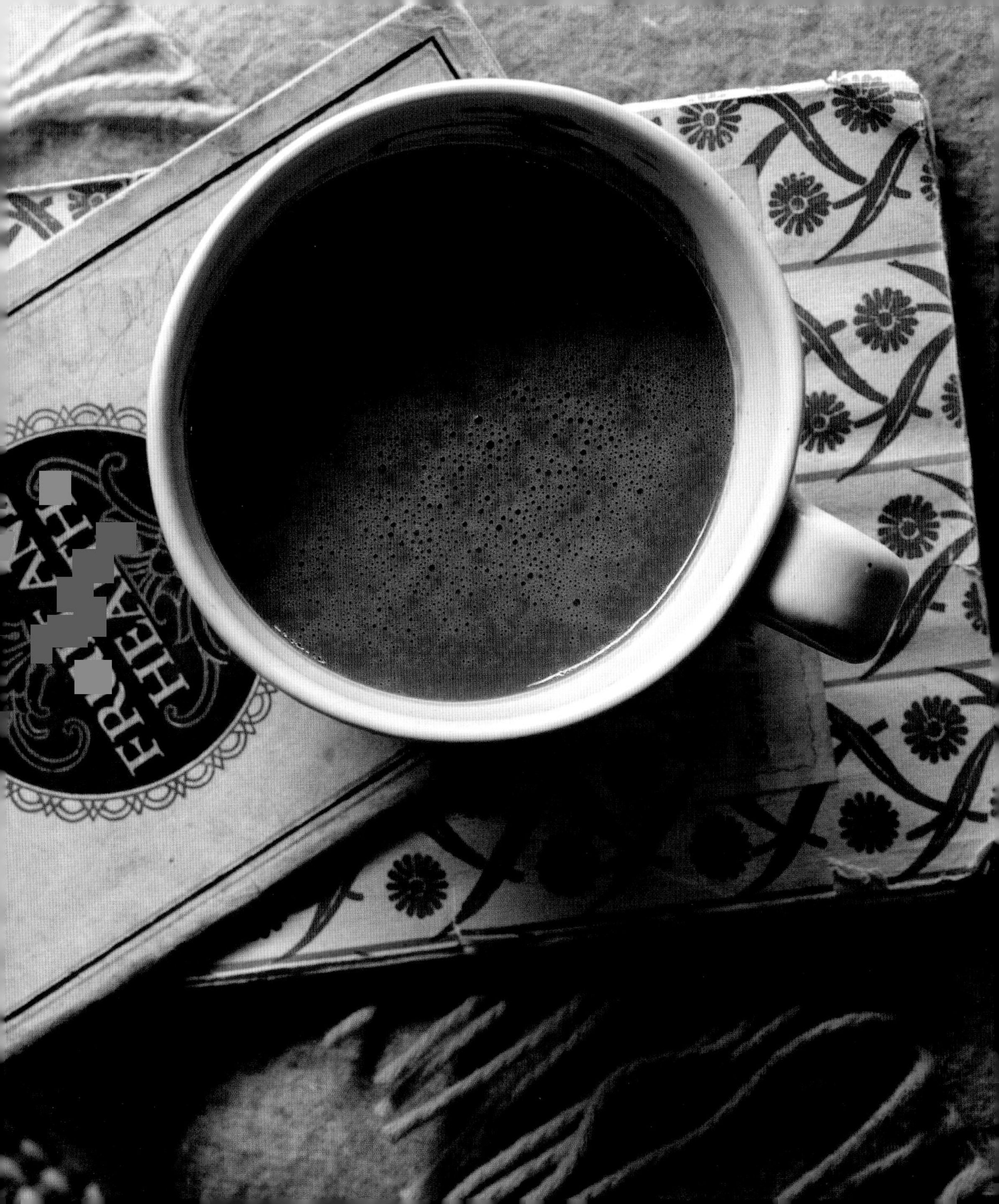

Warm milk with honey

SERVES 2
PREP: 5 minutes

480 ml / 16 fl oz soya or almond milk
1 cinnamon stick
a few drops of vanilla extract
1 tbsp clear honey
freshly grated nutmeg

A calming and relaxing warm milky drink gets you in the mood for bed and fosters a good night's sleep. The nutmeg has a natural sedative effect, inhibiting enzymes associated with stress; the honey contributes to melatonin release and the milk contains sleep-friendly tryptophan and vitamin D.

Put the soya or almond milk in a saucepan with the cinnamon stick and set over a medium heat. Heat very gently until the milk is really hot but don't let it boil.

Stir in the vanilla and honey and discard the cinnamon stick.

Pour into two mugs and grate some nutmeg over the top.

Or you can try this…

★ Top with a dusting of ground cinnamon.
★ Add some cardamom seeds with the cinnamon stick and strain the hot milk into the mugs.
★ Add half a teaspoon of ground turmeric.

Chamomile tea

Chamomile tea is an ancient and safe herbal remedy for insomnia. It is antibacterial and boosts the immune system, calms muscle spasms and aids digestion.

SERVES 2
PREP: 10 minutes
INFUSE: 5–10 minutes

2 tbsp fresh chamomile flowers
480 ml/16 fl oz water
honey for sweetening (optional)

Gently rinse the chamomile flowers in cold water to remove any dirt and insects.

Boil the water in a kettle and pour a little into a large china or earthenware teapot to warm it. Throw the water away.

Add the chamomile flowers to the warm pot and pour in the boiling water.

Cover the pot and leave to infuse for 5–10 minutes before straining into cups. If wished, stir in a little honey to sweeten the infusion.

Or you can try this ...

★ Add a sprig of mint or lemon verbena with the chamomile flowers.
★ Use chamomile teabags for a really quick cuppa – just follow the instructions on the packet.

Other teas to try ...

Chamomile, lavender and honey tisane

Combine some fresh lavender flowers with the chamomile flowers and infuse in boiling water for at least 5 minutes. Strain and sweeten with honey.

Lemon balm tea

Pour boiling water over some fresh lemon balm leaves or one tablespoon of dried lemon balm. Leave to infuse for at least 30 minutes before straining. Sweeten with honey if wished.

Index

Conversion tables

Conversions are approximate and have been rounded up or down.
Follow one set of measurements only – do not mix metric and imperial.

Weights

Metric	Imperial
15 g	½ oz
25 g	1 oz
40 g	1½ oz
50 g	2 oz
75 g	3 oz
100 g	4 oz
150 g	5 oz
175 g	6 oz
200 g	7 oz
225 g	8 oz
250 g	9 oz
275 g	10 oz
350 g	12 oz
375 g	13 oz
400 g	14 oz
425 g	15 oz
450 g	1 lb
550 g	1¼ lb
675 g	1½ lb
900 g	2 lb
1.5 kg	3 lb
1.75 kg	4 lb
2.25 kg	5 lb

Volume

Metric	Imperial
25 ml	1 fl oz
50 ml	2 fl oz
85 ml	3 fl oz
150 ml	5 fl oz (¼ pint)
300 ml	10 fl oz (½ pint)
450 ml	15 fl oz (¾ pint)
600 ml	1 pint
700 ml	1¼ pints
900 ml	1½ pints
1 litres	1¾ pints
1.2 litres	2 pints
1.25 litres	2¼ pints
1.5 litres	2½ pints
1.6 litres	2¾ pints
1.75 litres	3 pints
1.8 litres	3¼ pints
2 litres	3½ pints
2.1 litres	3¾ pints
2.25 litres	4 pints
2.75 litres	5 pints
3.4 litres	6 pints
3.9 litres	7 pints
5 litres	8 pints (1 gal)

Oven temperatures

140°C	275°F	Gas Mk 1
150°C	300°F	Gas Mk 2
160°C	325°F	Gas Mk 3
180°C	350°F	Gas Mk 4
190°C	375°F	Gas Mk 5
200°C	400°F	Gas Mk 6
220°C	425°F	Gas Mk 7
230°C	450°F	Gas Mk 8
240°C	475°F	Gas Mk 9